Use R!

T0203056

Series Editors:
Robert Gentleman   Kurt Hornik   Giovanni Parmigiani

Use R!

Roger D. Peng · Francesca Dominici

Statistical Methods for Environmental Epidemiology with R

A Case Study in Air Pollution and Health

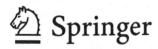 Springer

Roger D. Peng
Francesca Dominici
Johns Hopkins Bloomberg School
of Public Health
615 N. Wolfe St.
Johns Hopkins University
Baltimore MD 21205-2179
USA
rpeng@jhsph.edu
fdominic@jhsph.edu

Series Editors:
Robert Gentleman
Program in Computational Biology
Division of Public Health Sciences
Fred Hutchinson Cancer Research Center
1100 Fairview Avenue, N. M2-B876
Seattle, Washington 98109
USA

Kurt Hornik
Department of Statistik and Mathematik
Wirtschaftsuniversität Wien Augasse 2-6
A-1090 Wien
Austria

Giovanni Parmigiani
The Sidney Kimmel Comprehensive
Cancer Center at Johns Hopkins University
550 North Broadway
Baltimore, MD 21205-2011
USA

Library of Congress Control Number: 2008928295

ISBN 978-0-387-78166-2   ISBN 978-0-387-78167-9 (eBook)
DOI: 10.1007/978-0-387-78167-9

Printed on acid-free paper.

9 8 7 6 5 4 3 2 1

springer.com

Preface

As an area of statistical application, environmental epidemiology and more specifically, the estimation of health risk associated with the exposure to environmental agents, has led to the development of several statistical methods and software that can then be applied to other scientific areas. The statistical analyses aimed at addressing questions in environmental epidemiology have the following characteristics. Often the signal-to-noise ratio in the data is low and the targets of inference are inherently small risks. These constraints typically lead to the development and use of more sophisticated (and potentially less transparent) statistical models and the integration of large high-dimensional databases. New technologies and the widespread availability of powerful computing are also adding to the complexities of scientific investigation by allowing researchers to fit large numbers of models and search over many sets of variables. As the number of variables measured increases, so do the degrees of freedom for influencing the association between a risk factor and an outcome of interest.

We have written this book, in part, to describe our experiences developing and applying statistical methods for the estimation for air pollution health effects. Our experience has convinced us that the application of modern statistical methodology in a reproducible manner can bring to bear substantial benefits to policy-makers and scientists in this area. We believe that the methods described in this book are applicable to other areas of environmental epidemiology, particularly those areas involving spatial–temporal exposures.

In this book, we use the National Morbidity, Mortality, and Air Pollution Study (NMMAPS) and Medicare Air Pollution Study (MCAPS) datasets and describe the R packages for accessing the data. Chapters 4, 5, 6, and 7 describe the features of the data, the statistical concepts involved, and many of the methods used to analyze the data. Chapter 8 then shows how to bring all of the methods together to conduct a multi-site analysis of seasonally varying effects of PM_{10} on mortality.

A principal goal of this book is to disseminate R software and promote reproducible research in epidemiological studies and statistical research. As a case study we use data and methods relevant to investigating the health effects of ambient air pollution. Researching the health effects of air pollution presents an excellent example of the critical need for reproducible research because it involves all of the features already mentioned above: inherently small risks, significant policy implications, sophisticated statistical methodology, and very large databases linked from multiple sources. The complexity of the analyses involved and the policy relevance of the targets of inference demand transparency and reproducibility.

Throughout the book, we show how R can be used to make analyses reproducible and to structure the analytic process in a modular fashion. We find R to be a very natural tool for achieving this goal. In particular, for the production of this book, we have made use of the tools described in Chapter 3.

All of the data described in the book are provided in the **NMMAPSlite** and **MCAPS** R packages that can be downloaded from CRAN.[1] We have developed R packages for implementing the statistical methodology as well as for handling the databases. Packages that are not available from CRAN can be downloaded from the book's website.[2]

We would like to express our deepest appreciation to the many collaborators and students who have worked with us on various projects, short courses, and workshops that we have developed over the years. In particular, Aidan McDermott, Scott Zeger, Luu Pham, Jon Samet, Tom Louis, Leah Welty, Michelle Bell, and Sandy Eckel were all central to the development of the software, databases, exercises, and analyses presented in this book. Several anonymous reviewers provided helpful comments that improved the presentation of the material in the book. In addition, we would like to thank Duncan Thomas for many useful suggestions regarding an early draft of the manuscript. Finally, this work was supported in part by grant ES012054-03 from the National Institute of Environmental Health Sciences.

Baltimore, Maryland,   *Roger Peng*
April 2008   *Francesca Dominici*

---

[1] http://cran.r-project.org/
[2] http://www.biostat.jhsph.edu/~rpeng/useRbook/

Contents

1

Studies of Air Pollution and Health

1.1 Introduction

The material presented in this book is focused on statistical approaches for air pollution risk estimation in multi-site time series data, and specifically on the National Morbidity Mortality Air Pollution Study (NMMAPS). Because the datasets constructed as part of the NMMAPS include only publicly available data, the NMMAPS constitutes an ideal case study for illustrating the interdigitation among innovative statistical methods, their implementation in R, and software tools for reproducible research.

However, it is important to recognize that several other types of epidemiological studies have been introduced for estimating health effects of air pollution. Most of the air pollution epidemiological study designs have fallen into four types: ecological time series, case-crossover, panel, and cohort studies. Conceptually, panel studies collect individual time and space-varying outcomes, exposures, and confounders and therefore they encompass all other epidemiological designs which are based on spatially and/or temporally aggregated data. The time series, case-crossover, and panel studies are best suited for estimating the acute effects of air pollution, whereas cohort studies estimate acute and chronic effects combined. Acute effects are transient and due to time-varying exposures. Chronic effects are more likely due to the cumulative effects of exposure, but could be associated with more complex functions of lifetime exposure. Outcomes can be major or minor life events (e.g., death or onset of symptoms) or changes in function (e.g., vital capacity, lung growth, symptom severity). The nature of the outcome (e.g., binary, continuous, count, or time-to-event) and the structure of the data lead to the selection of the model and the types of effects to be estimated. Regression models are generally the method of choice.

This chapter is devoted to a brief description of each study design, identification of the corresponding approaches to statistical analysis, and presentation of examples. It concludes with a comparison of these designs.

1.2 Time Series Studies

Time series studies associate time-varying pollution exposures with time-varying event counts [7]. These are a type of ecologic study because they analyze daily population-averaged health outcomes and exposure levels. If the health effects are small and the disease outcomes are rare, the bias from ignoring the data aggregation across individuals should be small [122].

Generalized linear models (GLM) with parametric splines (e.g., natural cubic splines) [68] or generalized additive models (GAM) with nonparametric smoothers (e.g., smoothing splines or lowess smoothers) [45], are used to estimate effects associated with exposure to air pollution while accounting for smooth fluctuations in the mortality that confound estimates of the pollution effect.

The National Morbidity, Mortality and Air Pollution Study (NMMAPS) [35, 98, 101, 99, 27, 6, 77, 34] is the largest multisite time series study yet conducted. Unlike most other air pollution time series studies that concentrate on a single city, the goal of NMMAPS is to estimate city-specific, regional, and national effects of PM_{10} on mortality. Hierarchical models are particularly suitable for combining relative rates across locations. These methods and further NMMAPS results are discussed in the following sections of this book.

1.3 Case-Crossover Studies

The case-crossover design was originally proposed by Maclure [65] to study acute transient effects of intermittent exposures [48]. The case-crossover design can be viewed heuristically as a modification of the matched case-control design [8, 105] where each case acts as his or her own control, and the distribution of exposure is compared between cases and controls. More specifically, the exposure at the time just prior to the event (the *case* or *index time*) is compared to a set of *control* or *referent times* that represent the expected distribution of exposure for non-event follow-up times. In this way, the measured and unmeasured time-invariant characteristics of the subject (such as gender, age, smoking status) are matched, minimizing the possibility of confounding.

In the last decade of application, it has been shown that the case-crossover design is best suited to study intermittent exposures inducing immediate and transient risk, and abrupt rare outcomes [66, 48]. This design has been found to be topical for estimating the risk of a rare event associated with a short-term exposure to air pollution because the widespread availability of ambient monitoring data presents opportunities to further analyze existing case series from case-control studies.

Two main sources of potential bias in case-crossover studies have been identified and discussed in the literature [49, 50]. The first arises from the trend and seasonality in the air pollution time series. Because case-crossover comparisons are made within subjects at different points in time, the case-crossover analysis implicitly depends on the assumption that the exposure distribution is stationary. The long-term time trends and seasonal variation inherent in air pollution time series violate this assumption [73, 4, 64, 5, 60].

The second source of bias is called *overlap bias*. If the referent sets are exactly determined by the case period and are not disjoint, then the independent sampling inherent in the conditional likelihood approach is invalidated [1, 64]. Lumley and Levy [64] quantified the overlap bias analytically. Janes et al. [50] further explored the sources and magnitude of the overlap bias and concluded that the bias is usually small, although highly unpredictable and easily avoided.

The case-crossover design has been applied to many single studies of air pollution and health [111, 74, 81, 61, 22, 117] and to many multisite time series studies [126, 3, 2, 69] As an example Levy et al. [61] analyzed the effect of short-term changes in PM exposure on the risk of sudden cardiac arrest. The sample consisted of cases of paramedic-attended out-of-hospital primary cardiac arrest who were free of other life-threatening conditions and did not have a history of clinically detected cardiovascular disease. The cases were obtained from a previously conducted population-based case-control study and were combined with ambient air monitoring data. The results did not show any evidence of a short-term effect of PM air pollution on the risk of sudden cardiac arrest in people without previously recognized heart disease.

In a second example, Peters, et al. [82] conducted a case-crossover study in which cases of myocardial infarction were identified in Augsburg, in southern Germany, for the period from February 1999 to July 2001. There were 691 subjects for whom the date and time of the myocardial infarction were known who had survived for at least 24 hours after the event, completed the registry's standardized interview, and provided information on factors that may have triggered the myocardial infarction. Data on subjects' activities during the four days preceding the onset of symptoms were collected with the use of patient diaries. They found evidence that transient exposure to traffic may increase the risk of myocardial infarction in susceptible persons. The time the subjects spent in cars, on public transportation, or on motorcycles or bicycles was consistently linked with an increase in the risk of myocardial infarction.

1.4 Panel Studies

Panel studies enroll a cohort or panel of individuals and follow them over time to investigate changes in repeated outcome measures. They are most effective for studying short-term health effects of air pollutants, particularly in a susceptible subpopulation. Traditionally, a panel study design involves collecting repeat health outcome data for all N subjects over the entire time period of length T although this can be relaxed with proper accommodation in the analyses. The most suitable health outcomes vary within a person over the time period of observation. The pollution exposure measurement could be from a fixed-site ambient monitor, as well as personal monitors.

Studies that follow cohorts of individuals over longer time periods, say multiple years, are typically referred to as cohort or longitudinal studies rather than panel studies. Although the exposure and outcome characterization will be different, in general the recommended methods of analysis for longitudinal studies are similar to those developed for panel studies or cohort studies, depending upon the goals of the analyses.

The Southern California Children's Health Study [84, 83, 39] is one example of a longitudinal study of air pollution health effects. Children from grades 4, 7, and 10 residing in twelve communities near Los Angeles were followed annually. Communities were selected based on diversity in their historical air pollution levels. Longitudinal analyses of lung function growth using linear mixed models indicated associations of exposure to ambient particles, NO_2, and inorganic acid vapor with reduced lung function growth [39].

1.5 Cohort Studies

Air pollution cohort studies associate long-term exposure with health outcomes. Either a prospective or retrospective design is possible. In a prospective design, participants complete a questionnaire at entry into the study to elicit information about age, sex, weight, education, smoking history, and other subject-specific characteristics. They are followed over time for mortality or other health events. A measure of cumulative air pollution is often used as the exposure variable. A key design consideration for air pollution cohort studies is identifying a cohort with sufficient exposure variation. Individuals from multiple geographic locations must be studied in order to assure sufficient variation in cumulative exposure, particularly when ambient air pollution measurements are used. However, by maximizing the geographical variability of exposure, the relative risk estimates from cohort studies are likely to be confounded by area-specific characteristics.

Survival analysis tools can evaluate the association between air pollution and mortality. Typically the Cox proportional-hazards model [16, 14] is used to estimate mortality rate ratios for airborne pollutants while adjusting for potential confounding variables. Relative risk is estimated as the ratio of hazards for an exposed relative to an unexposed or reference group.

The epidemiological evidence on the long-term effects of air pollution on health has recently been reviewed by Pope [85]. The Harvard Six Cities study and the American Cancer Society (ACS) study [23, 89] are among the largest air pollution prospective cohort studies. In the Harvard Six Cities study [23, 57, 58] a random sample of 8111 adults who resided in one of the six U.S. communities at the time of the enrollment was followed for 14 to 16 years. An analysis of all-cause mortality revealed an increased risk of death associated with increases in particulate matter and sulfate air pollution after adjusting for individual-level confounders. Because of the small number of locations, findings of this study cannot be generalized easily.

The ACS study [89, 86, 87] evaluated effects of pollution on mortality using data from a large cohort drawn from 151 metropolitan areas. Ambient air pollution from these areas was linked with individual risk factors for 552,138 adult residents. The ACS study covered a larger number of areas, however, the subjects were not randomly sampled as in the Six Cities study. Both studies reported similar results: the relative risk of all-cause mortality was 1.26 (95% CI 1.08–1.47) for an 18.6 $\mu g/m^3$ change in fine particulate matter in the Six Cities study and 1.17 (95% CI 1.09–1.26) for a 24.5 $\mu g/m^3$ change in fine particulate matter in the ACS study. A detailed reanalysis of these two studies [56, 55] and a new ACS study including data for a longer period of time [86] replicated and extended these results by incorporating a number of new ecological covariates and applying several models for spatial autocorrelation.

1.6 Design Comparisons

Ultimately, the choice of an optimal design depends upon the research question and the availability of data. No single design is best for all applications. Each design targets specific types of effects, outcomes, and exposure sources. An optimal design should have sufficient power to detect the effect of exposure; this depends on the variability of exposure and the size of the study.

The panel and cohort studies can study events or continuous outcomes. Time series and case-crossover studies focus on events, and these events should be rare. One key difference between the time series and the case-crossover designs is the approach to control for seasonality and long-term time trends. The case-crossover study controls seasonality and trends by design through restriction of eligible referent samples. In contrast, time series studies use statistical adjustment in the regression model by including smooth functions of calendar time. In a recent paper Lu and Zeger [63] show that case-crossover using conditional logistic regression is a special case of time series analysis when there is a common exposure such as in air pollution studies. This equivalence provides computational convenience for case-crossover analyses and a better understanding of time series models. Time series log-linear regression accounts for overdispersion of the Poisson variance, whereas case-crossover analyses typically do not. This equivalence also permits model checking for case-crossover data using standard log-linear model diagnostics.

Acute effects can be estimated from panel, time series, and case-crossover studies. These studies rely exclusively on estimating associations between variation over time in exposure and variation over time in the outcome. Timescale analyses of time series studies [129, 109, 110, 30] allow estimation of such associations at different time scales: 1 month to 2 months, 1 to 2 weeks, 1 week to 3 days, and less than 3 days.

Cohort studies estimate a combination of acute and chronic effects because the outcomes accumulate over long time periods and could be triggered by either cumulative or short-term peak exposures. Thus, although estimation of chronic effects is one goal of cohort studies, these may not be separable from the acute effects of exposure [121, 23, 89, 56].

The effect of exposure may vary across susceptible subpopulations. The case-crossover, panel, and cohort study designs are better suited to directly assess effect modification across population groups than the time series design. The time series design aggregates events over a large population. Typically, individual risk factors or other information about the underlying population at risk is not available. In contrast, because each case is included individually in the analysis, the remaining three designs have the advantage of being able to target well-defined subgroups and to more directly evaluate personal characteristics as exposure effect modifiers.

2

Introduction to R and Air Pollution
and Health Data

2.1 Starting Up R

As of this writing the current version of R is version 2.7.0. In this book we make use of a number of R packages that do not come with the standard installation of R but are available elsewhere. The primary resource for obtaining R packages is the Comprehensive R Archive Network (CRAN) at

http://cran.r-project.org/

In addition to the main Web site, there are a number of mirrors located around the world which may provide faster access depending on the user's location.

Upon starting up R, the console prompt is presented to the user and commands can be input. The *workspace* can be thought of as an area of memory that can be used to store R objects or datasets. These objects are available until you quit R or they are deleted from the workspace. You can list the names of all the objects in the workspace by running

```
> ls()
```

```
character(0)
```

Currently, there are no objects in the workspace. Objects can be created via assignments, that is,

```
> x <- rnorm(10)
> print(x)
```

```
 [1]  1.89245635 -1.18982059 -0.01502809
 [4]  1.22581882  0.74902839 -0.17905201
 [7]  0.91236301  0.42186855 -0.62486494
[10]  0.73979867
```

and removed with the rm function.

```
> rm(x)
> ls()
```

```
character(0)
```

The entire workspace can be saved to a file using the save.image function. This saved workspace can subsequently be loaded back into R using the load function. The save function can be used to save individual objects in the workspace (as opposed to the entire workspace) to a file.

Packages can be loaded into an R session using the library function. Loading a package makes the exported functions in that package available to the user. The list of currently loaded packages can be seen with the search function.

```
> search()
```

```
[1] ".GlobalEnv"         "package:datasets"
[3] "package:utils"      "package:grDevices"
[5] "package:graphics"   "package:stats"
[7] "package:methods"    "Autoloads"
[9] "package:base"
```

R will load a number of packages by default when it starts up. The object named .GlobalEnv is meant to represent the user's workspace and it is always the first element of the search list

Two packages of which we make heavy use in this book are the **NMMAPSlite** package (described below in Section 2.3) and the **tsModel** package. These packages provide the datasets and statistical modeling code that we demonstrate throughout the book. All of the packages referenced in this book are available from CRAN or from the book's Web site. A CRAN package can be installed using the install.packages function. For example, to install the **NMMAPSlite** package, you can run in the console window

```
> install.packages("NMMAPSlite")
```

On most systems running this command will be sufficient. However, if you wish to install the package in another directory other than the default, you can run

```
> install.packages("NMMAPSlite", "mydirectory")
```

where mydirectory is the path to the library directory into which you want to install the package. Subsequently, you can load the package with the library function

```
> library(NMMAPSlite)
```

or

```
> library(NMMAPSlite, lib.loc = "mydirectory")
```

if you installed the package in a nonstandard directory.

2.2 The National Morbidity, Mortality, and Air Pollution Study

In this book we use as a running example and case study a large epidemiological study of the health effects of air pollution. The data consist of daily measurements of air pollution levels, meteorological variables, and mortality from various causes from over 100 cities in the United States. These data can be used for time series analyses of air pollution and mortality, a type of analysis that we describe in greater detail later on. Although the techniques that we describe are particularly useful for analyzing air pollution and health data, they are certainly applicable in other areas.

The National Morbidity, Mortality, and Air Pollution Study (NMMAPS) was a large national study of air pollution and health in the United States [98, 99, 101, 46]. The original study examined 90 major cities for the years 1987–1994, looking at mortality, hospitalizations, and the various ambient air pollution concentrations. The database for NMMAPS has recently been updated to include mortality and air pollution data for 108 cities spanning the years 1987–2000. Detailed information about the updated database is available on the Internet-based Health and Air Pollution Surveillance System (iHAPSS) Web site at

http://www.ihapss.jhsph.edu/

The NMMAPS database includes daily measurements on particulate matter (both PM_{10} and $PM_{2.5}$), ozone (O_3), sulphur dioxide (SO_2), nitrogen dioxide (NO_2), and carbon monoxide (CO). In our examples here we focus mainly on particulate matter and ozone. The pollution data were obtained from the Environmental Protection Agency's (EPA) Air Quality System (formerly known as the AIRS Database). Daily mortality data were compiled using death certificate data from the National Center for Health Statistics (NCHS). These data were aggregated into daily counts of mortality from various causes. Note that although the original NMMAPS examined hospitalization data from Medicare, these data are not included in the **NMMAPSlite** package or on the iHAPSS Web site.

2.3 Organization of the NMMAPSlite Package

Once all of the dependencies have been installed, the **NMMAPSlite** package can be installed and loaded into R in the usual way via library.

```
> library(NMMAPSlite)
> initDB("NMMAPS")
```

The **NMMAPSlite** package provides access to the NMMAPS data which reside on the iHAPSS server. The package itself does not contain any data, but rather provides functions for downloading the necessary data. The initDB function is called to indicate the directory in which the local cache of the NMMAPS database will be stored as it is downloaded from the iHAPSS repository. Here, we use the directory "NMMAPS" for the local cache.

The **NMMAPSlite** package provides access to data for 108 U.S. cities. All of the data in **NMMAPSlite** are split into three databases:

1. outcome: Daily time series of mortality for various causes and other data related to the outcomes. Each mortality time series is stratified into three age categories: under 65 years of age (under65), 65–74 (65to74), and 75 and older (75p). The mortality data are stored as an object of class "site".
2. exposure: Meteorological and pollution data stored as data frames.
3. Meta: Metadata pertaining to all the sites in the database.

The outcome, exposure, and Meta databases are key-value style databases stored in a format designated by the **stashR** package. For the outcome and exposure databases the key is the name of the city and value is the data frame associated with that city. Data can be loaded with the readCity function, which assigns the data being loaded to an R object. The metadata can be obtained from the Meta database using the getMetaData function.

2.3.1 Reading city-specific data

The data in **NMMAPSlite** are organized by city and each city's dataset can be accessed via its abbreviated name. To list all of the names available in the database, you can use the listCities function.

```
> cities <- listCities()
> head(cities, 20)

 [1] "akr"  "albu" "anch" "arlv" "atla" "aust"
 [7] "bake" "balt" "batr" "bidd" "birm" "bost"
[13] "buff" "cayc" "cdrp" "char" "chic" "cinc"
[19] "clev" "clmg"
```

To load a particular city's dataset, we can use the readCity function which has three arguments:

1. name, the abbreviated name of a city, passed as a character string
2. collapseAge, a logical indicating whether the three age categories into which the outcome data are split should be collapsed (default is FALSE)
3. asDataFrame, a logical indicating if readSite should return a data frame or not (default is TRUE)

If the asDataFrame argument to readSite is FALSE, readSite returns a list containing the outcome and exposure data frames. The list has two elements:

1. outcome, which contains a data frame of the mortality data by time and age category

2. exposure, a data frame containing daily time series of weather and air pollution variables

2.3.2 Pollutant data detrending

The pollutant data for each of the cities in the NMMAPS database has been processed in a manner that should be useful for the types of modeling we do in this book. This section gives a brief description of how the pollutant data series were constructed from the raw monitor data. For each city and pollutant, the basic algorithm shown below was followed.

1. Each city has associated with it a number of monitors for a given pollutant. The possible pollutants are PM_{10}, $PM_{2.5}$, SO_2, O_3, NO_2, and CO.
2. Let $X_{j,t}^c$ be the raw pollutant value for monitor j in city c at time/day t. The detrended value $\tilde{X}_{j,t}^c$ is defined as

$$M_{j,t}^c = \frac{1}{365} \sum_{\ell=-182}^{182} X_{j,t-\ell}^c$$

$$\tilde{X}_{j,t}^c = X_{j,t}^c - M_{j,t}^c$$

The values $\tilde{X}_{j,t}^c$ are the detrended "residuals" from the raw pollutant series and $M_{j,t}^c$ is a 365 day moving average for the pollutant.
3. If a city only has one monitor, then the series $\tilde{X}_{j,t}^c$ is the final result and can be used for analysis. Adding the series $\tilde{X}_{j,t}^c$ and $M_{j,t}^c$ gives back the original data.
4. If a city has two monitors, then a final $\bar{X}_t^c$ is computed for each time point t as

$$\bar{X}_t^c = \frac{1}{2}\left(\tilde{X}_{1,t}^c + \tilde{X}_{2,t}^c\right)$$

5. If a city has more than two monitors, then a 10% trimmed mean of the $\tilde{X}_{j,t}^c$s is taken for each day. That is, if there are J monitors in a city, then for each timepoint t,

$$\bar{X}_t^c = \text{TrimmedMean}_{10\%}\left[\tilde{X}_{1,t}^c, \ldots, \tilde{X}_{J,t}^c\right]$$

If there are fewer than ten monitors, the lowest and highest values for each day are still always discarded. One can see now why the detrending must be done first in Step 2. If a particular monitor has a higher overall level, then it will consistently be discarded when the trimmed mean is taken.
6. The series $\bar{X}_t^c$ is used as the pollutant measurement for city c on day t. In each city dataframe, this series is given the name *tmean where "*" is either pm10, pm25, so2, o3, no2, or co.

7. The median of the 365-day moving averages are also computed; that is,

$$\bar{M}_t^c = \text{Median}\left[M_{1,t}^c, \ldots, M_{J,t}^c\right]$$

This series is given the name *mtrend in each dataframe where "*" is the name of a pollutant. Adding the series $\bar{X}_t^c$ and $\bar{M}_t^c$ gives a series that resembles a standard pollutant series (rather than one centered around zero) but the series does not correspond to any particular monitor.

The data frames do not contain the original monitor data, but if one wishes to examine a series that is reminiscent of a true pollutant series, one can add the *tmean series to the *mtrend series. For example, to construct a PM$_{10}$ series, one can add the pm10tmean and pm10mtrend variables.

2.3.3 Mortality age categories

The mortality data are split into three age categories. For example, the data for New York City can be loaded as follows.

```
> site <- readCity("ny")
> site[1:5, 1:5]
```

```
          date accident copd cvd death
1 1987-01-01       10    3  22    73
2 1987-01-01        1    1  25    44
3 1987-01-01        2    2  66   105
4 1987-01-02        1    3  34    60
5 1987-01-02        2    3  80   118
```

Here, we show the first five rows and columns. Note above that the date "1987-01-01" appears three times. Because the mortality data are split over multiple strata (i.e., age categories), there is more than one mortality count per date of observation. If one is not interested in analyzing the mortality by age category, the argument collapseAge can be set to TRUE which aggregates the mortality counts across all strata.

```
> site <- readCity("ny", collapseAge = TRUE)
> site[1:5, 1:5]
```

```
          date accident copd cvd death
1 1987-01-01       13    6 113   222
2 1987-01-02        7   10 134   246
3 1987-01-03        5    3 123   214
4 1987-01-04        6    5 102   208
5 1987-01-05        4    6 114   228
```

2.3.4 Metadata

To see the full mapping between abbreviated city name and full city/state name, we can load some metadata for the cities. Metadata for the cities can be loaded using the getMetaData function. Called without arguments, getMetaData simply lists what metadata objects are available.

```
> getMetaData()

[1] "agecat"    "citycensus" "dow"
[4] "cities"    "counties"   "latlong"
[7] "regions"   "variables"  "siteList"
```

Metadata about each city are available in the citycensus object.

```
> census <- getMetaData("citycensus")
> head(census[, c("city", "pop100")])

  city pop100
1  akr 542899
2 albu 556678
3 amar 217858
4 anch 260283
5 arlv 189453
6 atla 1481871
```

Here we have listed the first few (abbreviated) city names and their respective populations. To find out which cities are available in the state of California, we can do

```
> cities <- getMetaData("cities")
> subset(cities, state == "CA", c(city,
+     cityname))

   city        cityname
7  bake       Bakersfield
33 fres            Fresno
49   la       Los Angeles
64 mode           Modesto
72 oakl           Oakland
84 rive         Riverside
86 sacr        Sacramento
89 sanb    San Bernardino
90 sand         San Diego
91 sanf     San Francisco
92 sanj          San Jose
96 staa Santa Ana/Anaheim
98 stoc         Stockton
```

The citycensus data frame contains much more information about each city obtained from the 2000 U.S. Census.

2.3.5 Configuration options

If the directory for storing the local cache of the database will be the same across multiple R sessions, it may be more convenient to set a user hook so that the appropriate directory is set automatically by initDB every time the **NMMAPSlite** package is loaded. One can do this by using the setHook function. For example, if we always wanted to use the "NMMAPS" directory to store the local cache, then we could call

```
setHook(packageEvent("NMMAPSlite", "onLoad"),
        function(...) NMMAPSlite::initDB("NMMAPS"))
```

This call to setHook could be placed, for example, in the user's .Rprofile file. Then, every time **NMMAPSlite** is loaded, the hook function is called and the directory for the local cache is automatically set.

2.4 MCAPS Data

The **MCAPS** package contains data and results related to the Medicare Air Pollution Study of Dominici et al. [33]. General information about the study can be found at

http://www.biostat.jhsph.edu/MCAPS/

This study was a multisite time series study of the short-term health effects of $PM_{2.5}$ in the United States. The study examined $PM_{2.5}$ and hospital admissions data from 204 U.S. counties for the period 1999–2002. The $PM_{2.5}$ data were obtained from the EPA's Air Quality System and the hospitalization data were obtained from Medicare. The study examined hospital admission for five cardiovascular outcomes, two respiratory outcomes, and injuries (as a sham outcome).

The **MCAPS** package contains maximum likelihood estimates and statistical variances of the county-specific log-relative risks of hospital admissions for each of the cardiovascular and respiratory diseases associated with lags 0, 1, and 2 exposure to $PM_{2.5}$. The package also contains air pollution and weather data used in the study. Figure 2.1 shows the locations of the 204 counties stratified by the seven geographical regions used.

The package can be loaded and initialized much the same way the **NMMAPSlite** package is loaded.

```
> library(MCAPS)
> initMCAPS("MCAPS")
```

Here, we use the directory MCAPS to store the local cache of the dataset. The objects that are available for download for this dataset can be listed by calling the getData function without arguments.

```
> getData()
```

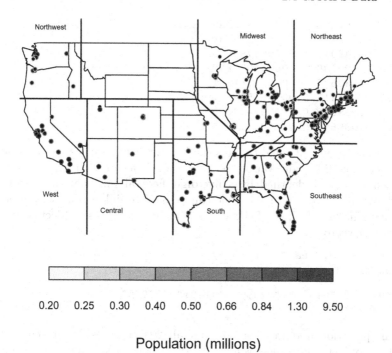

Population (millions)

Fig. 2.1. The 204 MCAPS counties, 1999–2002.

```
MCAPSinfo: APWdata, siteList,
estimates.subset, estimates.full
```

For example, the `estimates.subset` object is a data frame containing the maximum likelihood estimates of the log-relative risks for $PM_{2.5}$ and all eight outcomes for each county at the lag for which the largest association was found. (The `estimates.full` data frame contains the estimates for all lags.) We can obtain the estimated log-relative risks for heart failure by running

```
> estimates <- getData("estimates.subset")
> head(estimates[, c("CountyName", "outcome",
+     "beta", "var")])

      CountyName                    outcome
1 Jefferson, AL                      injury
2 Jefferson, AL cerebrovascular disease
3 Jefferson, AL      peripheral vascular
4 Jefferson, AL  ischemic heart disease
5 Jefferson, AL              heart rhythm
```

```
6 Jefferson, AL              heart failure
          beta                    var
1 -0.0006943051 0.000003799943
2  0.0011192680 0.000003080890
3 -0.0033530637 0.000010662981
4 -0.0007334413 0.000002514711
5  0.0012438399 0.000005624645
6  0.0014939658 0.000003996805
```

Here we show some of the estimates (and statistical variances) of the association between $PM_{2.5}$ and various outcomes for Jefferson County, Alabama.

Each county is identifed by a five-digit Federal Information Processing Standard (FIPS) code and this code can be used to link a county with other datasets. The list of all the FIPS codes is in the siteList object, which is a character vector.

```
> sites <- getData("siteList")
> head(sites)

[1] "01073" "01089" "01097" "01101" "02020"
[6] "04013"
```

The air pollution and weather data for all 204 counties are stored in the APWdata object. This object is a list of 204 data frames, one for each county; the list names are equal to the FIPS codes of the counties. Each data frame contains the following variables.

- date: the date in YYYY-MM-DD format
- pm25tmean: the trimmed mean of the $PM_{2.5}$ values across all monitors in the county
- tmpd: temperature (in degrees Fahrenheit)
- dptp: dewpoint temperature
- rmtmpd: a three-day running mean of temperature
- rmdptp: a three-day running mean of dew point temperature

For example, the Chicago data can be obtained by running

```
> apw <- getData("APWdata")
> chic <- apw[["17031"]]
> head(chic)

        date pm25tmean      tmpd dptp    rmtmpd
1 1999-01-01        NA 12.357143  7.7        NA
2 1999-01-02        NA 18.142857 21.0        NA
3 1999-01-03        NA 16.285714  8.4        NA
4 1999-01-04        NA  1.642857 -6.9 15.595238
5 1999-01-05        NA -2.000000 -6.1 12.023810
6 1999-01-06      23.9  8.142857  9.8  5.309524
      rmdptp
1         NA
```

```
2       NA
3       NA
4 12.366667
5  7.500000
6 -1.533333
```

3

Reproducible Research Tools

3.1 Introduction

The validity of conclusions from scientific investigations is typically strength-
ened by the replication of results by independent researchers. Full replication
of a study's results using independent methods, data, equipment, and proto-
cols, has long been, and will continue to be, the standard by which scientific
claims are evaluated. In many fields of study, there are examples of scientific
investigations that cannot be fully replicated, often because of a lack of time
or resources. For example, epidemiological studies that examine large populations and can potentially affect broad policy or regulatory decisions, often
cannot be fully replicated in the time frame necessary for making a specific
decision. In such situations, there is a need for a minimum standard that
can serve as an intermediate step between full replication and nothing. This
minimum standard is *reproducible research*, which requires that datasets and
computer code be made available to others for verifying published results and
conducting alternate analyses.

There are a number of reasons why the need for reproducible research is
increasing. Investigators are more frequently examining inherently weak associations and complex interactions for which the data contain a low signal-to-
noise ratio. New technologies allow scientists in all areas to compile complex
high-dimensional databases and the ubiquity of powerful statistical and computing capabilities allows investigators to explore those databases and identify
associations of potential interest. However, with the increase in data and computing power comes a greater potential for identifying spurious associations.
In addition to these developments, recent reports of fraudulent research being
published in the biomedical literature have highlighted the need for reproducibility in biomedical studies and have invited the attention of the major
medical journals [59].

Interest in reproducible research in the statistical community has been
increasing in the past decade [9, 94, 104]. The area of bioinformatics has

produced projects such as Bioconductor [42] which promotes reproducible research as a primary aim [see also 96, 41].

A proposal for making research reproducible in an epidemiological context was outlined in Peng et al. [78]. The criteria described there include a requirement that analytic data and the analytic computer code be made available for others to examine. The analytic data are defined as the dataset that served as the input to the analytic code to produce the principal results of the article. For example, a rectangular data frame might be analytic data in one case, a regression procedure might constitute analytic code, and regression coefficients with standard errors might be the principal results. Peng et al. [78] describe the need for reproducible research to be the minimum standard in epidemiological studies, particularly when full replication of a study is not possible.

The standard of reproducible research requires that the source materials of a scientific investigation be made available to others. This requirement is analogous to the definition of open source software,[1] which requires that the source code for a computer program be made available. However, by using the phrase "source materials" in the context of reproducible research, we do not mean simply the computer code that was used to analyze the data. Rather, we refer more generally to the preferred form for making modifications to the original analysis or investigation. Typically, this preferred form includes analytic datasets, analytic code, and documentation of the code and datasets.

The task of making research reproducible is not what one might consider a traditional statistical problem. However, statisticians are often confronted with the challenges of reproducing the computational results of others and statisticians are often the ones challenged with making their own results and computations reproducible by others. It is in this sense that we consider reproducible research a statistical problem for which we need to develop models and methods.

3.2 Distributing Reproducible Research

The distribution of reproducible research is a problem for which the solution varies depending on the complexity of the research. Small investigations involving moderately sized datasets and standard computational techniques can be archived and distributed in their entirety. Readers can subsequently rerun the entire analysis from start to finish to see if they can obtain the same results as the authors. Complex investigations involving large or multiple linked datasets and sophisticated statistical computations will be more difficult for readers to reproduce because of the resources and time required for running the analysis. In such a situation a method is needed to give readers without equivalent resources the ability to conduct an initial examination of the details of the investigation and to reproduce or verify some of the results.

---

[1] see, e.g., http://www.opensource.org/

A framework in which reproducible research can be distributed using *cached computations* is described in Peng and Eckel [79]. Cached computations are results that are stored in a database as an analysis is being conducted. These stored results can be distributed via Web sites or central repositories so that others may explore the datasets and computer code for a given scientific investigation.

We have developed some tools for assisting authors and researchers in conducting reproducible research and in writing reproducible packages. The R package that we describe here is the **cacher** package which provides tools for "caching" statistical analyses and for distributing these analyses to others in an efficient manner. Once distributed, a statistical analysis can be reproduced, modified, or improved upon. The **cacher** package is an implementation of the distributed reproducible research ideas described in Peng and Eckel [79].

At the end of each chapter in this book that contains substantial statistical analyses, we make reference to a cached package that the reader can download using the **cacher** package in order to reproduce any of the analyses in that chapter. The cached packages are hosted on the Reproducible Research Archive at http://penguin.biostat.jhsph.edu/. For example, in order to download the code and data for reproducing the analyses in chapter 5, the reader can execute

```
> clonecache(id = "2a04c4d5523816f531f98b141c0eb17c6273f308")
```

Partial matching is done with the package identifiers, so that

```
> clonecache(id = "2a04c4d")
```

would also download the code and data for chapter 5. This chapter demonstrates how to use the **cacher** package for exploring and verifying cached statistical analyses as well as caching one's own statistical analyses and distributing these analyses over the web.

3.3 Getting Started

To illustrate some of the features of the **cacher** package we use the following simple statistical analysis of the `airquality` dataset from the **datasets** package that comes with R. The code for the entire analysis is printed below.

```
library(datasets)
library(stats)

data(airquality)

fit <- lm(Ozone ~ Wind + Temp + Solar.R, data = airquality)
summary(fit)

## Plot some diagnostics
```

```
par(mfrow = c(2, 2))
plot(fit)

## Interesting nonlinear relationship
temp <- airquality$Temp
ozone <- airquality$Ozone

par(mfrow = c(1, 1))
plot(temp, ozone)
```

The code is contained in a file called "sample.R" that comes with the **cacher** package. The above analysis is fairly simple and not very time-consuming so it is easily reproduced by anyone who can run R, without any need for caching. Nevertheless, it is useful for demonstrating how the **cacher** package works.

The first step is to install the **cacher** package from the Comprehensive R Archive Network (CRAN) and load it into R.

```
> library(cacher)
> setConfig("verbose", TRUE)
```

For now, we also set the global verbose option to be TRUE, making cacher be somewhat more "chatty" (the default is FALSE).

3.4 Exploring a Cached Analysis

Once an analysis has been cached using cacher, it can be explored using the utilities provided in the **cacher** package. For example, we can download the analysis based on the "sample.R" file mentioned previously by calling

```
> clonecache(id = "44bf1c6e")
```

Because you can cache analyses from multiple files (as we have done here), we can show which analyses have already been cached using the showfiles function.

```
> showfiles()

[1] "sample.R"
```

If you want to examine an analysis, you can use the sourcefile function to choose that analysis and showcode will simply display the raw source file.

```
> sourcefile("sample.R")
> showcode()

library(datasets)
library(stats)

data(airquality)
```

```
fit <- lm(Ozone ~ Wind + Temp + Solar.R, data = airquality)
summary(fit)

## Plot some diagnostics
par(mfrow = c(2, 2))
plot(fit)

## Interesting non-linear relationship
temp <- airquality$Temp
ozone <- airquality$Ozone

par(mfrow = c(1, 1))
plot(temp, ozone)
```

You can also use the `code` function to display the code in a summary form.

```
> code()

source file: sample.R
1   library(datasets)
2   library(stats)
3   data(airquality)
4   fit <- lm(Ozone ~ Wind + Temp +
5   summary(fit)
6   par(mfrow = c(2, 2))
7   plot(fit)
8   temp <- airquality$Temp
9   ozone <- airquality$Ozone
10  par(mfrow = c(1, 1))
11  plot(temp, ozone)
```

The `code` function truncates expressions to a single line and also shows the sequence number assigned to each expression in the order that the expression is encountered in the source file. To see the full code for each expression, you can set the `full = TRUE` option to `code`.

The first thing you might do when exploring a cached analysis is to explore the elements of the cache database itself. You can list the objects available using the `showobjects` function, which returns a character vector of the names of each object in the database. Passing an expression sequence number to `showobjects` via the `num` argument shows the objects created by that expression.

```
> showobjects()

[1] "airquality" "fit"        "temp"
[4] "ozone"

> showobjects(8)

[1] "temp"
```

```
> showobjects(1)
```

```
character(0)
```

These objects can be lazy-loaded into the workspace using the `loadcache`
function.

```
> loadcache()
> ls()
```

```
[1] "airquality" "fit"          "ozone"
[4] "temp"
```

Now, we can print the linear model fit (without actually fitting the model) by
calling

```
> print(fit)
```

```
Call:
lm(formula = Ozone ~ Wind + Temp + Solar.R, data = airquality)
```

```
Coefficients:
(Intercept)         Wind          Temp
  -64.34208     -3.33359       1.65209
    Solar.R
    0.05982
```

The `loadcache` function takes a `num` argument which can be a vector of
indices indicating code expression sequence numbers. For example, if you want
to load only the objects associated with expression 4 (i.e., the `fit` object),
then you can call `loadcache(4)`.

In addition to exploring the objects in the cache database, you may wish
to run the analysis on your own computer for the purposes of reproducing the
original results. You can run individual expressions or a sequence of expressions with the `runcode` function. The `runcode` function accepts a number
or a sequence of numbers indicating expressions in an analysis. For example,
in order to run the first four expressions in the "sample.R" analysis, we could
call

```
> rm(list = ls())
> code(1:4)
```

```
source file: sample.R
1   library(datasets)
2   library(stats)
3   data(airquality)
4   fit <- lm(Ozone ~ Wind + Temp +
```

```
> runcode(1:4)
```

```
evaluating expression 1
evaluating expression 2
loading cache for expression 3
loading cache for expression 4

> ls()

[1] "airquality" "fit"
```

In this case, expressions 1 and 2 are evaluated but expressions 3 and 4 are loaded from the cache. By default, runcode does not evaluate expressions for which it can load the results from the cache. In order to force evaluation of all expressions, you need to set the option forceAll = TRUE.

3.5 Verifying a Cached Analysis

Once you have cloned an analysis conducted by someone else, you may wish to verify that the computation that you run on your computer leads to the same results that the original author obtained on her computer. This can be done with the checkcode function. The checkcode function essentially evaluates each expression locally (if it can) and compares the output with the corresponding value stored in the cache database.

If the locally created object and the cached object are the same, then that expression is considered verified. If an expression does not create any objects, then there is nothing to compare. If the locally created object and the cached object are different, the verification fails and checkcode will indicate which objects it could not verify.

For example, we can run the checkcode function on the analysis of the airquality dataset from before. Here we only check the first four code expressions.

```
> clonecache(id = "4eff7470")

created cache directory '.cache'
downloading source file list
downloading metadata
downloading source files
downloading cache database file list
downloading metadata
downloading source files
downloading cache database file list

> sourcefile("sample.R")
> showobjects(1:4)

[1] "airquality" "fit"

> checkcode(1:4)
```

```
evaluating expression 1
evaluating expression 2
checking expression 3
/ transferring cache db file 142d241ba5b4fbb564...
+ object 'airquality' OK
checking expression 4
/ transferring cache db file ad5720cbda29135e84...
+ object 'fit' OK
```

In the first four expressions, there are two objects created: the dataset airquality and the linear model object fit. The checkcode function compares each of those objects with the version stored in the cache database (which we previously cloned from the web). In this case, the objects match and the computations are verified. Notice that in expression 3, the database file for the airquality object had to be downloaded so that it could be checked against the locally created version.

Consider the following very simple analysis contained in the "bigvector.R" file that comes with the **cacher** package.

```
x <- rnorm(1000000)
s <- summary(x)
print(s)
```

We can check the code in the "bigvector.R" analysis also. In this analysis there are two objects that need to be verified: x, the vector of standard Normals and s the "summary" object.

```
> sourcefile("bigvector.R")
> checkcode()

checking expression 1
/ transferring cache db file fb877f8375799370ce...
- object 'x' not verified, FAILED
- Mean relative difference: 1.414514
checking expression 2
/ transferring cache db file d7952a4732ffa55c04...
- object 's' not verified, FAILED
- Mean relative difference: 0.0626853
evaluating expression 3
        Min.      1st Qu.      Median         Mean
-4.61500000 -0.67500000  0.00055530 -0.00002724
     3rd Qu.        Max.
 0.67460000   5.02200000
```

Notice that expressions 1 and 2 failed for a common reason (expression 3 had no objects to verify). Because the analysis did not set the random number generator seed in the beginning, the generation of the Normal random variates on the local machine is not the same as that for the original analysis. Therefore, the object x is not reproducible (nor is s).

Of course, there are limitations to verifying statistical analyses. Analyses may take a long time to run and therefore it may take a long time to verify a given computation. If one does not have the necessary external resources (i.e. hardware, software) then it may not be possible to verify an analysis at all. Currently, verification of analyses is limited to R objects only. We cannot verify the output of summary or print functions nor can we verify plots (although lattice plots can be verified if they are stored as R objects).

Certain analyses may load external datasets or inputs that will generally not be available to the other users. A typical analysis might be of the form

```
data <- read.csv("faithful.csv")
with(data, plot(waiting, eruptions))

library(splines)
fit <- lm(eruptions ~ ns(waiting, 4), data = data)

xpts <- with(data, seq(min(waiting), max(waiting), len = 100))
lines(xpts, predict(fit, data.frame(waiting = xpts)))
```

This analysis reads in the the "Old Faithful" dataset which contains eruption times and waiting periods for the Old Faithful geyser in Yellowstone National Park. Although this dataset is available from the R installation, we have exported it here to a comma-separated-value file for demonstration.

The original author of this analysis can run the `cacher` function on this analysis file and distribute it to others.

```
> cacher("faithful.R")
```

However, another user (presumably on a different computer) will not be able to verify all of the code in this analysis

```
> sourcefile("faithful.R")
> checkcode()

checking expression 1
- problem evaluating expression, FAILED
- simpleWarning: cannot open file
- 'faithful.csv': No such file or directory
- loading objects from cache
/ transferring cache db file 255fb954f855b0e53b...
evaluating expression 2
evaluating expression 3
checking expression 4
/ transferring cache db file a15033591616f8a9b6...
+ object 'fit' OK
checking expression 5
/ transferring cache db file bed8272d401434750a...
+ object 'xpts' OK
evaluating expression 6
```

Here, the first expression, which reads the dataset in via read.csv cannot be verified because the "faithful.csv" file is not available. However, the other expressions can be run on the local machine and are verifiable because they can use the cached copy of the dataset.

3.6 Caching a Statistical Analysis

An author can cache an analysis once it is completed and distribute it over the Web using the facilities in the **cacher** package. The cacher function accepts a file name as its first argument. This file should contain the code for the analysis that you want to cache. Other arguments include the name of the cache directory (defaults to .cache) and the name of the log file (defaults to NULL). If logfile = NULL then messages will be printed to a file in the cache directory. Setting logfile = NA will send messages to the console.

The "sample.R" file containing the above analysis comes with the **cacher** package and can be copied into your working directory. Given a file containing the code of an analysis, you can call the cacher function as

```
> cacher("sample.R")

Call:
lm(formula = Ozone ~ Wind + Temp + Solar.R, data = airquality)

Residuals:
    Min      1Q  Median      3Q     Max
-40.485 -14.219  -3.551  10.097  95.619

Coefficients:
             Estimate Std. Error t value
(Intercept) -64.34208   23.05472  -2.791
Wind         -3.33359    0.65441  -5.094
Temp          1.65209    0.25353   6.516
Solar.R       0.05982    0.02319   2.580
                 Pr(>|t|)
(Intercept)       0.00623 **
Wind      0.00000151593 ***
Temp      0.00000000242 ***
Solar.R           0.01124 *
---
Signif. codes:  0 '***' 0.001 '**' 0.01 '*' 0.05 '.' 0.1 ' ' 1

Residual standard error: 21.18 on 107 degrees of freedom
  (42 observations deleted due to missingness)
Multiple R-squared: 0.6059, Adjusted R-squared: 0.5948
F-statistic: 54.83 on 3 and 107 DF,  p-value: < 2.2e-16
```

The cacher function evaluates each expression in the file and prints any resulting output to the console. For example, the summary of the fitted linear model is printed to the console and the two plots are sent to the appropriate graphics device.

3.7 Distributing a Cached Analysis

If you have access to a Web server you can post your cache directory directly on the Web server for others to access. Once made available on a Web server, others can access your cache directory by using the clonecache function in the **cacher** package and the URL of the directory on your Web server. For example, we can download the analysis corresponding to the "bigvector.R" file by calling

```
> clonecache
    ("http://www.biostat.jhsph.edu/rr/bigvector.cache")

created cache directory '.cache'
downloading source file list
downloading metadata
downloading source files
downloading cache database file list
```

This call to clonecache downloads all of the relevant cache files related to the analysis except for the cache database files. In order to download the cache database files, the option all.files = TRUE must be set.

Once a cache package has been downloaded using clonecache you can use all of the tools described in the previous sections to explore the cache and then run some of the analyses.

```
> showfiles()

[1] "bigvector.R"

> sourcefile("bigvector.R")
> code()

source file: bigvector.R
1   x <- rnorm(1000000)
2   s <- summary(x)
3   print(s)

> showobjects()

[1] "x" "s"

> loadcache()
> print(s)

/ transferring cache db file d7952a4732ffa55c04...
        Min.    1st Qu.     Median        Mean
-4.6570000 -0.6737000  0.0006063  0.0012460
     3rd Qu.       Max.
 0.6755000  5.1400000
```

By default, clonecache does not download the cache database files until
they are needed in order to minimize the amount of data that is transferred.
Cache database files are only transferred from the remote host when the objects associated with them are first accessed.

In the above example, the database file corresponding to the object s is
only transferred when we call print(s). When a database object has to
be downloaded from the remote site, a message will be printed to the screen
indicating the transfer.

3.8 Summary

Using the **cacher** package, authors can cache an analysis and distribute the
analysis over the Web in a standard format. The **cacher** package also provides
readers tools for downloading these cached analyses and exploring the code
and data within them. Readers can selectively download R objects for inspection and for reproducing parts of an analysis. In addition, tools are provided
for verifying the computations in an analysis so that readers can be sure that
their calculations match those of the original authors.

Chapters 5, 6, 7, and 8 all have cache packages associated with them and
at the end of each chapter we describe how to download those packages to
reproduce the analyses. In addition, Section 7.2 of Chapter 7 gives a complete
demonstration of how to use the **cacher** package to reproduce one of the
MCAPS analyses.

4

Statistical Issues in Estimating the Health Effects of Spatial–Temporal Environmental Exposures

4.1 Introduction

Statistical methods for environmental processes are typically centered around the idea of building a model that can produce good predictions of the process itself based on a chosen criterion. For example, in a typical spatial statistics problem we might be concerned with predicting the mean value of a process in an unobserved location conditional on the observed data.

However, when analyzing air pollution and health data, we are primarily interested in estimating and understanding the association between an exposure to an environmental agent and an outcome. For example, we may be interested in understanding the relationship between day-to-day changes air pollution levels and day-to-day changes in mortality counts. We are not interested in predicting the mortality count for any given day. In the end, we would like to "tell a story" about the relationship between an exposure and a health outcome. The more information we have with which to tell that story, the better.

Our goals of examining the relationships between environmental exposures and health events and of summarizing the evidence from the data lead us to a subtle but distinctly different statistical focus. We largely eschew predictive models and model-building techniques based on optimizing predictive accuracy and precision. Rather, we focus on methods that allow us to estimate certain parameters of interest and allow us to understand uncertainty due to adjustment for potential confounders, as opposed to traditional model uncertainty. In summary, we need useful statistical models for estimating associations rather than for prediction.

In this chapter we focus on the features of temporal data that allow us to build good statistical models and to ultimately estimate the health effects of environmental exposures accounting for all the sources of uncertainty.

4.2 Time-Varying Environmental Exposures

The statistical methods described in this book will be relevant to the analysis of spatially or temporally varying environmental agents of interest that might affect human health. An important aspect of many environmental exposures is that repeated measurements are taken over time and/or space. This book in particular examines more carefully environmental exposures that vary in time and which are most often represented as *time series* data.

Figure 4.1(a) shows a time series of daily levels of particulate matter less than 10 μm (PM_{10}) from Salt Lake City, Utah for the years 1998–2000. In Figure 4.1(b) we have the corresponding daily time series of nonaccidental mortality for the same city and time period. These data were taken from the National Morbidity, Mortality, and Air Pollution Study (NMMAPS) database, a large multicity air pollution and mortality database [99, 101]. Specifically, the **NMMAPSlite** package described in Chapter 2 was used to retrieve the city data.

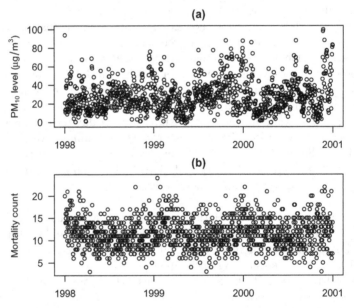

Fig. 4.1. (a) Daily PM_{10} levels and (b) daily nonaccidental mortality counts in Salt Lake City, Utah, 1998–2000.

The data for both mortality and PM_{10} exhibit variation on a number of different timescales, with seasonal patterns as well as day-to-day variability. We use these variations on different timescales to illustrate our approach to displaying the evidence of association between PM_{10} and mortality in the next sections.

4.3 Estimation Versus Prediction

One question of scientific interest might be, "Are changes in the PM_{10} series associated with changes in the mortality series?" This question is fundamentally about the relationship between a time-varying health outcome y_t and a time-varying exposure x_t. A simple linear model might relate

$$y_t = \beta_0 + \beta_1 x_t + \varepsilon_t \tag{4.1}$$

where β_0 is the mean mortality count, β_1 is the increase in mortality associated with a unit increase in PM_{10}, and ε_t is a stationary mean zero error process. Such a model certainly describes the association between y_t and x_t: a positive value of β_1 might indicate evidence of an adverse affect of PM_{10} whereas a zero or negative value might indicate that there is a "protective" effect or, more likely, that something else is going on. For example, in model (4.1) we have omitted any variables that might explain the covariation in x_t and y_t. These *potential confounders* might produce a negative estimate of β_1 if they are omitted from the model. This is an important issue to which we return later.

Although model (4.1) appears to serve a useful purpose, perhaps we can do a little better. For example, suppose we took the exposure series x_t and decomposed it into two parts,

$$x_t = \bar{x}_t^Y + (x_t - \bar{x}_t^Y)$$

where $\bar{x}_t^Y$ is a yearly two-sided moving average of PM_{10} and $(x_t - \bar{x}_t^Y)$ is the deviation of the current value from that yearly average. Using the above decomposition of x_t, we can reformulate (4.1) to get

$$y_t = \beta_0 + \beta_1 \bar{x}_t^Y + \beta_2 (x_t - \bar{x}_t^Y) + \varepsilon_t \tag{4.2}$$

Note that model (4.2) is equivalent to model (4.1) if $\beta_1 = \beta_2$, however, model (4.2) does not require them to be equal. Furthermore, model (4.2) produces the same predictions as model (4.1).

We can continue along these lines by letting $z_t = x_t - \bar{x}_t^Y$ and decomposing z_t as

$$z_t = \bar{z}_t^S + (z_t - \bar{z}_t^S)$$

where $\bar{z}_t^S$ is a three-month moving average of z_t, representing the seasonal variation in the z_t series. Now we can use the model

$$y_t = \beta_0 + \beta_1 \bar{x}_t^Y + \beta_2 \bar{z}_t^S + \beta_3 (z_t - \bar{z}_t^S) + \varepsilon_t \tag{4.3}$$

Going one step further, let $u_t = z_t - \bar{z}_t^S$ and decompose

$$u_t = \bar{u}_t^W + (u_t - \bar{u}_t^W)$$

where $\bar{u}_t^W$ is a weekly moving average of u_t. Let $r_t = (u_t - \bar{u}_t^W)$ represent the residual variation in the time series. Then our expanded model is now

$$y_t = \beta_0 + \beta_1 \bar{x}_t^Y + \beta_2 \bar{z}_t^S + \beta_3 \bar{u}_t^W + \beta_4 r_t + \varepsilon_t \qquad (4.4)$$

We have now decomposed the original exposure series x_t into four separate components representing the yearly, seasonal, weekly, and sub-weekly/daily variation in the PM_{10} data. In particular, note that we have preserved the relationship

$$x_t = \bar{x}_t^Y + \bar{z}_t^S + \bar{u}_t^W + r_t$$

Why is such a decomposition of x_t useful? First, model (4.4) includes model (4.1) as a special case (where $\beta_1 = \beta_2 = \beta_3 = \beta_4$) so we have not lost any information. Rather, we have gained information because with model (4.4) each of the parameters $\beta_i, i = 1, \ldots, 4$ relates changes in x_t to changes in y_t over different timescales.

For example, β_1 describes the association between y_t and the yearly average of x_t. We might expect this parameter to be large because a unit increase in the yearly average of PM_{10} represents a fairly large change in pollution levels for a location. However, we must use caution here because the relationship between y_t and the yearly average of x_t could easily be confounded by other factors in a location that vary smoothly over time. For example, long-term changes in the population size could affect long-term trends in both pollution levels and mortality counts. Similarly, general improvements in technology might decrease overall levels of pollution as well as mortality.

The parameter β_4 describes the association between y_t and the sub-weekly fluctuations in x_t (adjusted for the yearly, seasonal, and weekly variation). We might expect β_4 to be small relative to β_1 because a unit change in PM_{10} over the course of a few days does not represent such a dramatic change in pollution levels as does a unit change in the yearly average. In addition, the factors that might confound an estimate of β_1 would likely not affect our estimate of β_4. However, care must still be taken in interpreting β_4 which can be affected by other factors that vary at similar short-term timescales. One notable example is temperature, which can be correlated with particular pollutants such as ozone and PM_{10} as well as with daily mortality.

An important task for the statistician and the substantive expert is to identify what might confound the relationship between y_t and x_t at the different timescales. We have given some examples for the yearly and the subweekly timescales but there are potentially more. The decomposition in model (4.4) allows us to divide the task of identifying potential confounders into separate compartments.

The feature of time series exposure data that we have highlighted here is the possibility of breaking the time axis into meaningful subdivisions or groupings, what we call timescales. We can look at yearly, quarterly, monthly, or weekly averages and differences from those averages. These natural subdivisions aid us in interpretation and can help us to more usefully categorize the effects of potential confounders.

Each of models (4.1)–(4.4) produces the same predictions of the outcome y_t. If we were solely interested in predicting the outcome, then it would not be of any added benefit to introduce this timescale decomposition. However, because we are interested in "telling a story" about y_t and x_t, it is useful to decompose the exposure variable so that we can see from where the evidence of an association comes. With model (4.4) we have a richer descriptive model with which to make decisions about potential confounding and can more fully understand the relationship between y_t and x_t. In Section 5.3 we provide some examples on how to estimate the association between y_t and x_t at each timescale of temporal variation in the data.

4.4 Semiparametric Models

The previous section showed how with time series data the exposure can be decomposed into different timescales to aid us in interpreting the relationship between the outcome y_t and the exposure x_t. One important issue that we did not discuss in the previous section is how to deal with the effects of other factors that may confound the relationship between y_t and x_t. The framework of *semiparametric models* will allow us to simultaneously adjust for the effects of multiple potential confounders (including time) while still benefiting from the timescale decomposition in a slightly different manner.

Whenever we examine the relationship between a health outcome and an exposure, we must be wary of other factors that might confound the relationship between the two. Often we have corresponding data for those factors and can adjust for them directly in a statistical model. For example, when looking at PM_{10} and mortality, one important variable to consider is the weather, which can affect both pollution levels and mortality. Many cities have meterological measurements such as temperature, dewpoint temperature, and humidity so that if we take those variables as an approximation of the "weather", then we can adjust for them directly in the models.

No matter how many measurements we have on other factors that might confound the relationship between y_t and x_t, there will always remain the possibility of there being yet another confounding factor that is unmeasured. In time series models, the factors about which we are most concerned are factors that vary in time in a manner similar to air pollution and health outcomes. When we have data on these factors we can attempt to adjust for them directly in models. However, when data are not available, we must resort to a proxy for those factors.

In a semiparametric linear model we can attempt to adjust for unmeasured time-varying potential confounders by using a smooth function of time itself. If y_t is the response and x_t is the exposure, then we can fit a model of the form

$$y_t = \alpha + \beta x_t + \boldsymbol{\eta}' \mathbf{z}_t + f(t; \lambda) + \varepsilon_t$$

where β is the risk coefficient of interest, $\mathbf{z}$ is a vector of measured covariates that we want to adjust for directly in the model, and $f(t; \lambda)$ is the smooth function of time. The behavior of f is controlled by the smoothing parameter λ, which can be thought of as the degrees of freedom allowed for f. Larger values of λ imply a rougher f function wherease smaller values of λ imply a smoother function.

Air pollution studies commonly involve count data as the response (i.e., daily mortality or hospitalization counts), in which case we can use a Poisson generalized linear model of the form

$$Y_t \sim \text{Poisson}(\mu_t)$$
$$\log \mu_t = \alpha + \beta\, x_t + \boldsymbol{\eta}' \mathbf{z}_t + f(t; \lambda) + \varepsilon_t \tag{4.5}$$

where μ_t is the mean response for day t and β is the log-relative risk associated with the exposure x_t.

There have been many different proposals in the literature regarding how f should be represented and fit to the data, including using natural splines, penalized splines, smoothing splines, and loess. In addition to the representation issue is the question of how smooth or rough should f be. Again, there have been numerous methods developed for determining the optimal smoothness for f. The various advantages and disadvantages of using these methods are discussed in detail in [76].

4.4.1 Overdispersion

In the previous Section 4.4 we made the assumption that $Y_t \sim \text{Poisson}(\mu_t)$, implying that $\text{var}(Y_t) = \mu_t$. This assumption can be easily relaxed by introducing an overdispersion parameter ϕ, such that $\text{var}(Y_t) = v_t = \phi\mu_t$. In this way, we are allowing the counts Y_t to have variances v_t that might exceed their means μ_t (i.e., be overdispersed) with overdispersion parameter ϕ. In practice, after having fitted the semiparametric (4.5) allowing for overdispersion, we will often find that the estimated ϕ is close to one. This is likely due to the fact that, by including a smooth function of time in (4.5), we are removing most of the residual outcorrelation in the data. A data analysis example where we allow for overdispersion is presented in Section 6.6.4.

4.4.2 Representations for f

Two common choices for representing the smooth function f are natural (cubic) splines and penalized splines. Natural splines are piecewise cubic polynomials defined on a grid of knot locations spanning the range of the data. The function itself, as well as its second derivative, is continuous on the entire range of the data and the function is restricted to be linear beyond the endpoints. The smoothness of a natural spline fit is controlled by the number of knots used. Fewer knots represent smoother fits and a large number of knots will lead to data interpolation. The knot locations are typically chosen to be at regressor values associated with equally spaced quantiles but could be anywhere.

Penalized splines provide an alternate way to model nonlinear relationships. They have been presented in the literature in a number of ways and we use the general definition $\hat{\boldsymbol{\eta}}' \mathbf{B}(x)$, where

$$\hat{\boldsymbol{\eta}} = \arg\min_{\boldsymbol{\eta}} \sum_{i=1}^{n} \left\{ y_i - \boldsymbol{\eta}' \mathbf{B}(x_i) \right\}^2 + \alpha \boldsymbol{\eta}' \mathbf{H} \boldsymbol{\eta}.$$

$\mathbf{B}(x)$ is a spline basis matrix (evaluated at the point x), α is a penalty (smoothing) parameter, and $\mathbf{H}$ is a penalty matrix. Variations of penalized splines essentially boil down to different specifications of the spline basis matrix $\mathbf{B}$ and the form of the penalty $\mathbf{H}$. Typically, one constructs a natural spline or B-spline basis using a large number of knots and then shrinks the coefficients to reduce the effective degrees of freedom and increase smoothness in the overall function estimate [67, 124]. The amount of smoothness in the estimated curve is controlled by α. As $\alpha \downarrow 0$, the amount of smoothing decreases; as $\alpha \uparrow \infty$, the amount of smoothing increases and the estimated curve approaches a polynomial function.

The most extreme approach to knot placement in the penalized spline framework is to place the maximum number of knots possible, that is, one knot at every data point. The resulting fit is then called a smoothing spline. Time series data are typically regularly spaced and the smoothing spline scheme leads to n equally spaced knots along the time period of the dataset. Because smoothing splines can be considered a special case of penalized splines [95], results obtained using smoothing splines should be similar to those obtained using penalized splines.

The complexity of a spline basis representation can be measured by its degrees of freedom. Natural splines, penalized splines, and smoothing splines all give rise to linear smoothers, thus they can be represented by the $n \times n$ smoother matrix that maps the observed data to the predicted values. The effective degrees of freedom are computed by the trace of the smoother matrix [10, 45]. For fully parametric fits such as those using natural splines, this trace equals the number of estimated parameters in the model.

4.4.3 Estimation of β

For the purposes of this section, we focus on the estimation of β and the smooth function of time f. Using matrix notation, we can rewrite (4.5) as

$$\begin{aligned} \mathbf{Y} &\sim \text{Poisson}(\boldsymbol{\mu}) \\ \log \boldsymbol{\mu} &= X\beta + \mathbf{f} \end{aligned} \tag{4.6}$$

where $\mathbf{Y} = y_1, \ldots, y_n$, $\mathbf{f}$ is the function f evaluated at $t = 1, \ldots, n$, and X is the $n \times 2$ design matrix containing a column of ones and the pollution time series $x_1, \ldots, x_n$.

Given an $n \times d$ spline basis matrix B, we can rewrite (4.6) as

$$\log \boldsymbol{\mu} = X\boldsymbol{\beta} + B\boldsymbol{\gamma}$$

where γ is a d-vector of coefficients. The number of columns of the basis matrix B will be different depending on whether natural splines, penalized splines, or smoothing splines are used.

We use iteratively reweighted least squares (IRLS) to fit model (4.6) using natural splines. Let W be the $n \times n$ (diagonal) weight matrix and $\mathbf{z}$ the working response from the last iteration of the IRLS algorithm. Let X^* be the complete design matrix (i.e., $X^* = [X \mid B]$). The estimates of β and γ are

$$\begin{bmatrix} \widehat{\beta}_{ns} \\ \widehat{\gamma} \end{bmatrix} = (X^{*'}WX^*)^{-1}X^{*'}W\mathbf{z}$$

For penalized splines, we first need to construct the smoother matrix for the nonparametric part of the model. Given a value for the smoothing parameter α and a fixed (symmetric) penalty matrix H, the smoother matrix for $\mathbf{f}$ is

$$S = B(B'B + \alpha H)^{-1}B'$$

and the estimate of β is

$$\widehat{\beta}_{ps} = (X'W(I - S)X)^{-1}X'W(I - S)\mathbf{z}$$

It is important to note that the use of natural splines and penalized splines to represent the smooth function f should not be considered interchangeable methods. For example, Rice [92] and Speckman [113] both showed that although the variance of $\widehat{\beta}_{ps}$ converges at the standard parametric rate for $n \to \infty$, the bias converges to zero at the much slower nonparametric rate. The slow convergence of the bias comes from the fact that the smoother matrix S is not a true projection, unlike the hat matrix in parametric regression [113].

4.4.4 Choosing the degrees of freedom for f

Given a particular representation of f described in Section 4.4.2, one must then choose the degrees of freedom (df) controlling the amount of smoothness allowed for f. A general strategy is to use a data-driven method and select a df that optimizes a particular criterion. For example, one approach is to choose the df that leads to optimal prediction of the health outcome series and another is to select the df that best predicts the pollution series. With each of these approaches, a number of Poisson regression models are fit using a range of df values (other covariates such as weather variables and the pollutant variable are included). Then, for each fitted model, a model selection criterion is evaluated with the "optimal" df being that which minimizes the criterion. In multisite studies, this approach can lead to a different df selected for each location, potentially allowing location-specific characteristics of the data to influence the estimated smoothness of f.

Theoretical analysis has shown that choosing the degrees of freedom that allows the smooth function of time to best predict the pollution series x_t leads to an estimate of the β that is asymptotically unbiased [28]. Subsequent simulation studies have generally agreed with the theoretical findings and have shown choosing the df to best predict the pollution series leads to estimates with small bias, particularly when the true f and x_t are highly correlated [76].

An alternate approach is to use a fixed degrees of freedom, perhaps based on biological knowledge or previous work. For multisite studies, this approach leads to fitting the same model to data from each location. One can explore the sensitivity of $\widehat{\beta}$ by varying the df used in the model(s) and examining the associated changes in $\widehat{\beta}$.

4.5 Combining Information and Hierarchical Models

One of the recent statistical advances in the study of short-term effects of air pollution on health has been the use of hierarchical models to combine information from multiple counties or cities. Such multisite studies have provided strong evidence of a short-term association between PM_{10} and mortality. The combining of information not only increases the power and precision of estimates but it can protect those results from the uncertainty due to model adjustments for potential confounders. We explore the use of hierarchical models in much greater detail in Chapter 7, but we outline the basic principles here.

Suppose we have data for multiple cities and those cities are indexed by $c = 1, \ldots, n$. Then one possible approach we can take is to estimate a location-specific log-relative risk $\hat{\beta}^c$ using a semiparametric model such as the one described in Section 4.4. Along with the location-specific risk estimates, we can estimate a location-specific variance $\hat{\sigma}_c^2$ for that risk estimate. The variance estimates $\hat{\sigma}_c^2$ can be thought of as the "within-location" statistical uncertainty associated with $\hat{\beta}^c$.

In all likelihood, the estimates $\hat{\beta}^c$ will differ from location to location over a range of values. One explanation of the variation in risk estimates might be that those cities are different from each other and have very different qualities and therefore should exhibit different risks. Another possibility is that although the risk estimates are different, they only appear so because of the noise in the data and the uncertainty of the estimates themselves. We can use an hierarchical model to attempt to separate out what might be "true" variation between cities and what might simply be the noise. A simple model assumes

$$\hat{\beta}^c \mid \beta^c \sim \mathcal{N}(\beta^c, \hat{\sigma}_c^2)$$

and

$$\beta^c \sim \mathcal{N}(\mu, \tau^2).$$

Here, the estimated location-specific risk estimates $\hat{\beta}^c$ are assumed to be Normally distributed around an unknown "true" risk estimate β^c with variance $\hat{\sigma}_c^2$. Then, the true risk estimates are assumed to be Normally distributed around an overall average μ with variance τ^2. The parameter τ^2 is sometimes referred to as the *heterogeneity* variance.

In some cases we may be interested in examining posterior estimates of the location-specific risk estimates that borrow information from other locations. We can produce the shrunken estimates β^c as the posterior mean of the distribution

$$\beta^c \mid \hat{\beta}^c \sim \mathcal{N}\left(\mu + \frac{\tau^2}{\hat{\sigma}_c^2 + \tau^2}(\hat{\beta}^c - \mu), \frac{\hat{\sigma}_c^2 \tau^2}{\hat{\sigma}_c^2 + \tau^2}\right)$$

The use of an hierarchical model involves making specific assumptions about the nature of variation in the location-specific estimates across locations. For example, the Normal distribution used here allows the β^cs to be negative, which may or may not be plausible depending on the specific application. In addition, another assumption that is typically made is the independence of estimates from different locations. Of course, hierarchical models are only useful when data for multiple locations are in fact available. In particular, the estimation of the heterogeneity variance τ^2 depends critically on there being enough locations to estimate the variation of the "true" log-relative risks across locations.

5

Exploratory Data Analyses

5.1 Introduction

What do time series data look like? The purpose of this chapter is to provide a number of different answers to this question. In addition, we outline the rudiments of a time series analysis of air pollution and mortality that can be used to connect the two to look for interesting relationships.

5.2 Exploring the Data: Basic Features and Properties

5.2.1 Pollutant data

The NMMAPS database has information about six of the criteria pollutants defined by the United States Environmental Protection Agency. These pollutants are measured by the EPA's monitoring network and the raw data are available on the EPA's Air Quality System Web site. In this section we describe some of the features of the pollutant data.

Particulate matter

For illustration, we begin with the Baltimore, Maryland data.

```
> balt <- readCity("balt", asDataFrame = FALSE)
```

The air pollution and weather data are stored in a data frame called "exposure". The PM_{10} time series in particular is stored in a variable named "pm10tmean".

```
> with(balt$exposure, summary(pm10tmean))
     Min.   1st Qu.   Median     Mean   3rd Qu.
 -35.1300  -10.7200  -3.1500  -0.1274    7.5330
     Max.      NA's
  94.8700 3173.0000
```

There are a number of interesting features of the PM_{10} data here. First, notice the large number of missing values (NAs) in this particular variable. The time series contains daily data for 14 years (January 1, 1987 through December 31, 2000), which means the total length of the series (including missing values) is 5114. Of those 5114 possible values, 3173 of them are missing. The reason for this is that PM_{10} measurements are only made once every three days in Baltimore. So for every three days of potential measurement, two are always missing. For the later years, the sampling pattern is changed to be one in six days, so there are even more missing values for those years. Most cities in the U.S. have this kind of sampling pattern for PM_{10} data, although there are a handful of cities with daily measurements.

Another feature is that the mean and median are close to zero. How can there be negative PM_{10} values one might wonder? Each of the pollutant time series have been detrended so that they are roughly centered about zero. Details of the detrending can be found in [101] and in Chapter 2. Generally speaking, the detrending does not have a big impact on potential analyses because in time series studies we are primarily interested in differences from day to day, rather than differences between mean levels. If one is interested in reconstructing approximately the original values, the "median trend" is stored in a variable called "pm10mtrend" and can be added to the "pm10tmean" variable.

```
> with(balt$exposure, summary(pm10tmean +
+      pm10mtrend))

    Min.    1st Qu.    Median     Mean    3rd Qu.
  0.5449   21.2300   28.6000   32.1900    40.0800
    Max.      NA's
130.5000  3173.0000
```

Another aspect worth noting about the pollutant data is that air pollution concentrations in the NMMAPS database are averaged across multiple monitors in a given city. When multiple monitor values are available for a given day, a 10% trimmed mean is taken to obtain the value stored in the database (hence the "tmean" part of the variable name).

We can plot the data to examine some more features. The resulting plot is shown in Figure 5.1.

```
> with(balt$exposure, {
+      plot(date, pm10tmean + pm10mtrend,
+           ylab = expression(PM[10]), cex = 0.6)
+ })
```

One thing that is clear from the time plot of the data in Figure 5.1 is that the variability of PM_{10} has decreased over the 14 year period. After about 1995, we do not see the same number of very high values as we do before 1995. Note that here we have plotted the PM_{10} data with the trend added back in

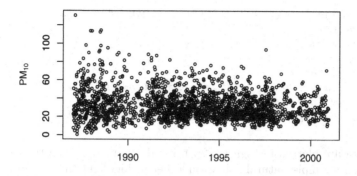

Fig. 5.1. PM_{10} data for Baltimore, Maryland, 1987–2000.

so that we can examine the long-term trends in PM_{10}. To look at the trend more formally, we can conduct a simple linear regression of PM_{10} and time.

```
> library(stats)
> pm10 <- with(balt$exposure, pm10tmean +
+      pm10mtrend)
> x <- balt$exposure[, "date"]
> fit <- lm(pm10 ~ x)
```

The table of regression parameter estimates is shown in Table 5.1. The negative slope parameter indicates a downward linear trend in PM_{10}. If we look

	Estimate	Std. Error	t value	$Pr(>|t|)$
(Intercept)	47.8966	2.3076	20.76	0.0000
x	−0.0018	0.0003	−6.89	0.0000

Table 5.1. Regression analysis of long-term trend in PM10.

more closely at a few years, we can see more patterns and trends. In particular, we can examine differences in these patterns across locations. Here, we plot the Baltimore, Maryland PM_{10} data for the years 1998–2000.

```
> subdata <- subset(balt$exposure, date >=
+      as.Date("1998-01-01"))
> subdata <- transform(subdata, pm10 = pm10tmean +
+      pm10mtrend)
> fit <- lm(pm10 ~ ns(date, df = 2 * 3),
+      data = subdata)
```

```
> x <- seq(as.Date("1998-01-01"), as.Date("2000-12-31"),
+     "week")
> par(mar = c(2, 4, 2, 2), mfrow = c(2,
+     1))
> with(subdata, {
+     plot(date, pm10, ylab = expression(PM[10]),
+         main = "(a) Baltimore", cex = 0.8)
+     lines(x, predict(fit, data.frame(date = x)))
+ })
```

These data are plotted in Figure 5.2(a). In addition to plotting the data, we
have added a simple natural spline smoother to highlight the overall trends.
The smoother uses two degrees of freedom per year of data to capture the
seasonality. There is a clear seasonal pattern in the PM_{10} data in Figure 5.2(a),

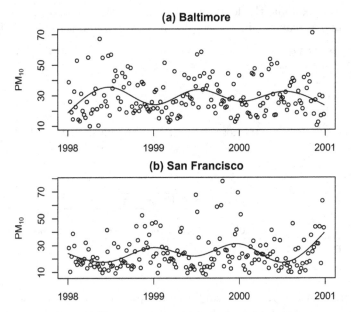

Fig. 5.2. PM_{10} data for (a) Baltimore, Maryland, and (b) San Francisco, California,
1998–2000.

where the summer days tend to have higher levels than the winter days.

The Baltimore PM_{10} data exhibit a common pattern among eastern U.S.
cities, which is a summer increase in PM_{10} levels and a winter decrease. The
pattern in the western United States is somewhat different. We can take a
look at data from San Francisco, California for the same three year period.

```
> sanf <- readCity("sanf", asDataFrame = FALSE)
> subdata <- subset(sanf$exposure, date >=
+     as.Date("1998-01-01"))
```

```
> subdata <- transform(subdata, pm10 = pm10tmean +
+     pm10mtrend)
> fit <- lm(pm10 ~ ns(date, df = 2 * 3),
+     data = subdata)
> x <- seq(as.Date("1998-01-01"), as.Date("2000-12-31"),
+     "week")
> with(subdata, {
+     plot(date, pm10, ylab = expression(PM[10]),
+         main = "(b) San Francisco", cex = 0.8)
+     lines(x, predict(fit, data.frame(date = x)))
+ })
```

The seasonal pattern for San Francisco in Figure 5.2(b) on the west coast is the exact opposite of the pattern exhibited for Baltimore on the east coast. Here, we have winter peaks in PM_{10} and summer lows. It is useful to note these patterns when we examine the mortality data in the next section.

Ozone

Another pollutant that is of great interest to many researchers is ozone (O_3) which has been linked to mortality and morbidity in various parts of the world [e.g., 6, and references therein]. Ozone is a gas that can form primarily but is usually a result of secondary interactions with other gases and sunlight. In particular, the formation of ozone is closely related to local meteorology. In many locations ozone is not measured during the fall and winter months because of the generally lower levels during that time.

Not every city in the NMMAPS database has ozone measurements. Here we look at the Baltimore and Chicago data. Ozone is measured in parts per billion (ppb) and has hourly measurements. The **NMMAPSlite** package has the hourly measurements for ozone for each day as well as an aggregate measure for the entire day. The variable o3tmean is a daily time series of the trimmed mean of the detrended 24-hour average of ozone. The trend for this series is stored in the variable o3mtrend.

We plot the ozone data for Baltimore and Chicago in Figure 5.3(a, b).

```
> balt <- readCity("balt", asDataFrame = FALSE)
> chic <- readCity("chic", asDataFrame = FALSE)

> par(mfrow = c(2, 1), mar = c(3, 4, 2,
+     2))
> with(balt$exposure, plot(date, o3tmean +
+     o3mtrend, main = "(a) Baltimore",
+     ylab = expression(O[3] * " (ppb)"),
+     pch = "."))
> with(chic$exposure, plot(date, o3tmean +
+     o3mtrend, main = "(b) Chicago", ylab = expression(O[3] *
+     " (ppb)"), pch = "."))
```

One can see immediately that ozone, like PM_{10}, is highly seasonal, here with a summer peak and winter trough in both cities. Baltimore has a different sampling pattern than Chicago in that for Baltimore there are only measurements between the six months of April through October.

In the United States, when ozone is measured it tends to be measured every day, so we do not have the kinds of missing data problems that we have with particulate matter. Ozone tends to be missing in a seasonal way, as with Baltimore, or sporadically. This pattern of missingness is also present with the other gases: sulphur dioxide, nitrogen dioxide, and carbon monoxide.

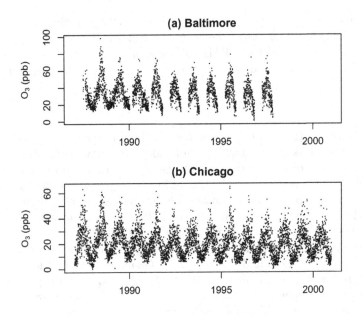

Fig. 5.3. Daily ozone data for (a) Baltimore and (b) Chicago, 1987–2000

5.2.2 Mortality data

The mortality data are stored in a separate element in the list returned by `readCity`. That element is named "outcome" and consists of a data frame. For the NMMAPS data, the outcomes consist of daily mortality counts starting from January 1, 1987 through December 31, 2000. The mortality counts are split into a number of different outcomes including mortality from all causes excluding accidents, chronic obstructive pulmonary disease (COPD), cardiovascular disease, respiratory disease, and accidents. Each mortality count series has an associated "mark" series of the same length which is 1 or 0 depending on whether a given day's count is seemingly outlying. One may wish to exclude very large counts in a given analysis and the "mark" variables are meant to assist in that.

The mortality data are also stratified into three age categories: mortality for people under age 65, age 65 to 74, and age over 75. The "outcome" object has a slot named "strata" which is a data frame containing factors indicating the different strata for the outcome data. In this case there is only one factor variable (agecat) indicating the three age categories. Lastly, the "outcome" object contains a "date" slot which is a vector of class "Date" indicating the date of each observation.

The outcome data for New York City can be read in via readCity. Here we have extracted the outcome data frame only. We can plot the mortality count for all-cause mortality by age group to see the different trends and seasonal patterns.

```
> data.split <- split(outcome, outcome$agecat)
> par(mfrow = c(3, 1), mar = c(2, 4, 2,
+     2) + 0.1)
> with(data.split[[1]], plot(date, death,
+     main = "Under 65", ylab = "Mortality count",
+     pch = "."))
> with(data.split[[2]], plot(date, death,
+     main = "65 to 74", ylab = "Mortality count",
+     pch = "."))
> with(data.split[[3]], plot(date, death,
+     main = "Over 75", ylab = "Mortality count",
+     pch = "."))
```

The mortality data for the three age categories are shown in Figure 5.4. Notice in Figure 5.4 that the three age categories have slightly different trends in mortality. The under 65 group appears to have a decreasing trend, particularly after 1995. The 64–75 group appears to have a more gradual decrease trend over the 14 year period and the over 75 group has a relatively stable trend in mortality. All groups have a strong seasonal pattern with a peak in winter and a trough in summer. The seasonality seems to be most pronounced in the over 75 group. The peak in winter mortality is most likely due to the spread of infectious diseases such as influenza as well as temperature-related phenomena in cold weather areas. Most important for subsequent health-related analyses, aside from temperature, data related to the causes of these seasonal changes in mortality are largely unavailable or unmeasured.

We can examine other features of the data such as the autocorrelation structure. With time series data such as these, we would expect that neighboring values (in time) would be more similar than distant values. One such tool for examining this behavior is the autocorrelation function, or acf. The acf is defined as [13]

$$r(k) = \frac{1}{N} \sum_{t=1}^{N-k} (x_t - \bar{x})(x_{t+k} - \bar{x})/c(0)$$

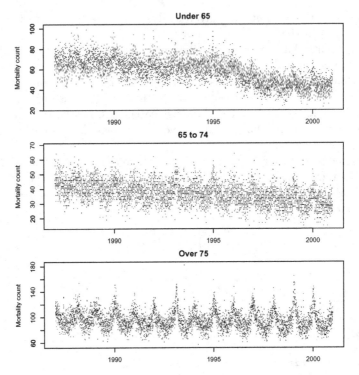

Fig. 5.4. New York City daily mortality data by age category, 1987–2000

where

$$c(0) = \frac{1}{N} \sum_{t=1}^{N} (x_t - \bar{x})^2$$

The integer k indicates the lag of the variable. A plot of $r(k)$ for $k = 0, 1, \dots, K$ is called a correlogram. Figure 5.5(a) shows a correlogram for the New York City mortality data. The correlogram can be computed in R using the `acf` function in the **stats** package.

```
> library(stats)
> par(mfrow = c(2, 1))
> x <- with(subset(outcome, agecat == "75p"),
+     death)
> acf(x, lag.max = 50, main = "(a) New York City mortality",
+     ci.col = "black")
```

The very slow decrease in autocorrelation from lag 1 to lag 50 shown in the plot indicates that there is some nonstationarity in the series. We can remove this by regressing the values of the series against a smooth function of time. This smooth function of time can be estimated using natural splines or possibly other nonparameteric methods. Here we use a natural spline smoother for simplicity.

```
> library(splines)
> fit <- lm(x ~ ns(1:5114, 2 * 14))
> xr <- resid(fit)
> label <- "(b) New York City mortality (seasonality removed)"
> acf(xr, lag.max = 50, main = label, ci.col = "black")
```

Figure 5.5(b) shows the correlogram of the residuals after removing some of the seasonality. There remains some autocorrelation but substantially less than that exhibited before the seasonality was removed. Season is an important

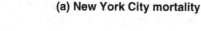

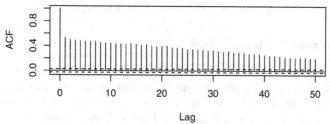

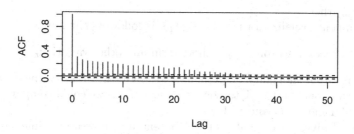

Fig. 5.5. Autocorrelation functions for New York City mortality data for (a) raw data and (b) residuals after removing seasonality.

variable to consider because as shown in Figures 5.4 and 5.2, season is related very strongly to both mortality and air pollution.

5.3 Exploratory Statistical Analysis

In many time series analyses, one is often interested in how a single variable, such as temperature, PM_{10}, or mortality, varies over time. We might be interested in how that variable varies from day to day, month to month, season to season, or year to year. The particular timescale of interest depends on the type of scientific question one is interested in addressing.

We may also be interested in examining how two variables co-vary with each other over time. Such questions may come in the form of, "If X increases today, does Y also increase today?" or, "If X increases this month, does Y increase next month?"

In the previous section, we examined individual variables and how they varied over time. We noticed that both PM_{10} and mortality have strong seasonal patterns and long-term (generally decreasing) trends. In this section we look at the relationship between mortality and PM_{10} and also examine what other variables might potentially confound that relationship.

5.3.1 Timescale decompositions

Common to all time series data is that we have values that vary over a time index. In the case of air pollution and mortality data, we have values that change from day to day. However, we may also be interested in timescales of variation beyond the day-to-day changes. For example, we may be interested in looking at the overall 14 year long-term trend of mortality or the seasonal behavior of PM_{10}. In such cases, it is useful to decompose the time series into separate components so that we can examine them separately rather than mix them all together.

We can conceptualize a time series $\{Y_t\}$ as following the model

$$Y_t = \text{trend}_t + \text{seasonality}_t + \text{short-term and other variation}_t \qquad (5.1)$$

where Y_t is either mortality or perhaps PM_{10}. Given access to the separate timescale components (trend, seasonality, short-term) we could compare them separately for mortality and PM_{10}.

Table 5.2 gives a schematic of the potentially interesting timescales in which we may be interested when examining air pollution and mortality. The three timescales for each variable are labeled generally as "Trend" for trends spanning across years, "Seasonal" for within-year patterns, and "Short-Term" for shorter-term fluctuations. Although we are interested in the timescale decompositions of both mortality and pollution separately, we are more interested in looking at how the two variables correlate at different timescales and in determining what kind of evidence is provided by such correlations.

Timescale decompositions of this kind are common in time series analysis. One example is the STL decomposition of [15] which is implemented in R in the `stl` function of the **stats** package. Cleveland's STL uses the nonparameteric smoother loess to decompose a time series into three separate components. Another possibility is to compute the Fourier transform of the time series and group the different frequency components together into trend, seasonal, and short-term components. The use of the Fourier transform allows for more precise examination of timescales beyond those already mentioned.

	Mortality		
	Trend	Seasonal	Short-Term
Trend	X		
Pollution Seasonal		X	
Short-Term			X

Table 5.2. Example timescales of interest for air pollution and health studies and the correlations between timescales of interest (marked with Xs)

One question that is useful to ask is how are mortality and air pollution levels correlated at each of the three different timescales?

In particular, we are potentially interested in estimating the correlations between the respective long-term trends of mortality and pollution, the seasonal trends, and the short-term fluctuations (the Xs marked in Table 5.2). Hence, the cells of interest in Table 5.2 are the ones falling on the diagonal. Although it is possible to look at other correlations in the table, their interpretation is less clear.

A related question one needs to ask is what might confound the relationship between mortality and air pollution at different timescales? For example, long-term decreases in PM_{10} might be positively correlated with long-term decreases in mortality, indicating that lowering air pollution levels is beneficial. However, there might be factors explaining both decreases, such as changes in population demographics and community-level activity patterns. Weather, and specifically temperature, is a factor that can confound the relationship between mortality and pollution at both the seasonal timescale and the short-term timescale because it too has seasonal trends and short-term flucutations. As with all correlation analyses, any evidence of association at a given timescale must be interpreted in the context of what might potentially confound that association.

5.3.2 Example: Timescale decompositions of PM_{10} and mortality

We use data from Detroit, Michigan to demonstrate the timescale decomposition introduced in the previous section. Here, we use the full 14 year daily time series available from the NMMAPS database and not the shortened series shown in Figure 4.1.

We decompose the time series data into three different timescales using moving averages as defined in Section 4.3. Because our method of using moving averages does not work well with missing values in the exposure variable, we will fill in the missing values with the mean of the entire series. There are only 52 missing values out of 5114 observations, thus this filling-in procedure does not have an impact on the results.

A simple linear regression of y and x gives us the results in Table 5.3.

```
> library(NMMAPSlite)
> library(stats)
> initDB("NMMAPS")
> data <- readCity("det", collapseAge = TRUE)
> y <- data[, "death"]
> x <- with(data, pm10tmean + pm10mtrend)
> dates <- data[, "date"]
> x[is.na(x)] <- mean(x, na.rm = TRUE)
> fit <- lm(y ~ x)
```

	Estimate	Std. Error	t value	Pr($>$|t|)
(Intercept)	46.1798	0.2263	204.11	0.0000
x	0.0232	0.0057	4.06	0.0000

Table 5.3. Simple linear regression of PM10 and mortality

There appears to be strong evidence of a positive association between PM_{10} and mortality. We can conduct a full timescale decomposition of the PM_{10} data to obtain a more detailed picture of the relationship between mortality and PM_{10} in Detroit.

```
> library(stats)
> x.yearly <- filter(x, rep(1/365, 365))
> z <- x - x.yearly
> z.seasonal <- filter(z, rep(1/90, 90))
> u <- z - z.seasonal
> u.weekly <- filter(u, rep(1/7, 7))
> r <- u - u.weekly
```

Upon decomposing the data, we can fit the model in (4.4) to obtain estimates of the yearly, seasonal, weekly, and sub-weekly associations.

```
> fit <- lm(y ~ x.yearly + z.seasonal +
+        u.weekly + r)
```

All of the timescales appear strongly associated with mortality. However, the seasonal component has a strong negative association. This is because Detroit's PM_{10} levels tend to be higher in the summer season and lower in the winter. In contrast, mortality is generally higher in the winter and lower in the summer. This inverse relationship gives us the negative coefficient for the seasonal component.

We can also produce a timescale decomposition of the mortality data and then plot the different timescales for mortality and PM_{10} next to each other to

	Estimate	Std. Error	t value	Pr($>|t|$)
(Intercept)	34.1031	1.3098	26.04	0.0000
x.yearly	0.3783	0.0383	9.88	0.0000
z.seasonal	−0.4354	0.0295	−14.76	0.0000
u.weekly	0.0532	0.0123	4.33	0.0000
r	0.0215	0.0070	3.07	0.0022

Table 5.4. Linear regression of PM10 and mortality, full decomposition

check for any interesting relationships. First we can decompose the mortality time series in to the same yearly, seasonal, weekly, and sub-weekly timescales.

```
> y.yearly <- filter(y, rep(1/365, 365))
> yz <- y - y.yearly
> yz.seasonal <- filter(yz, rep(1/90, 90))
> yu <- yz - yz.seasonal
> yu.weekly <- filter(yu, rep(1/7, 7))
> yr <- yu - yu.weekly
```

Figure 5.6 shows a portion of the timescale decompositions for the Detroit PM_{10} (left column) and daily mortality data (right column) for the years 1988–2000. Data are shown for the period 1988–2000 because we use the first year of data to calculate the moving averages. We can see a little more clearly the strong positive association between the yearly trends and the negative association between the seasonal components. The less smooth weekly and residual/subweekly components are difficult to examine by eye and we must resort to linear regression results in those cases.

5.3.3 Correlation at different timescales: A look at the Chicago data

Dominici et al.[29] provided software for creating timescale decompositions of time series data via a Fourier transform. We have packaged their software and have included it in the **tsModel** package. The tsdecomp function can be used to decompose a time series into user-specified timescales. We demonstrate the use of tsdecomp on mortality and PM_{10} data from Chicago, Illinois.

```
> data <- readCity("chic", collapseAge = TRUE)
> death <- data[, "death"]
> is.na(death) <- as.logical(data[, "markdeath"])
```

The Chicago mortality data contain a few days with extremely high mortality counts. Although these may be of interest in another analysis, they are outliers with respect to the other data points and we remove them for the time being by setting them to be NA. The variable markdeath is an indicator of days that have outlying mortality counts.

First we can identify important characteristics of the mortality data by decomposing the series into three different timescales. The timescales include

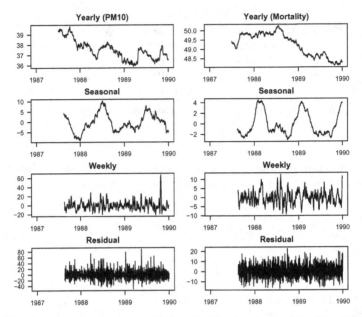

Fig. 5.6. Timescale decomposition for Detroit PM_{10} and mortality data, 1987–2000.

- A single cycle over the entire series
- 2–14 cycles over the entire series
- 15 or more cycles

These timescales correspond roughly to long-term trends, seasonal trends, and higher frequency short-term trends.

```
> library(tsModel)
> mort.dc <- tsdecomp(death, c(1, 2, 15,
+     5114))
```

The three time scales are plotted in Figure 5.7.

```
> par(mfrow = c(3, 1), mar = c(3, 4, 2,
+     2) + 0.1)
> x <- seq(as.Date("1987-01-01"), as.Date("2000-12-31"),
+     "day")
> plot(x, mort.dc[, 1], type = "l", ylab = "Trend",
+     main = "(a)")
> plot(x, mort.dc[, 2], type = "l", ylab = "Seasonal",
+     main = "(b)")
> plot(x, mort.dc[, 3], type = "l", ylab = "Residual",
+     main = "(c)")
```

Figure 5.7(a) shows the long-term trend which is generally decreasing, not unlike the trend observed with the New York City mortality data. Here we have collapsed the three age categories and are examining the aggregated series. Figure 5.7(b) shows the obvious seasonal pattern in the mortality data, again with a winter peak and summer trough. Figure 5.7(c), the bottom plot, shows the residual variation in mortality, once the long-term trend and seasonality have been removed. Note that the original series is equal to the sum of the three plots in Figures 5.7(a–c). A similar timescale decomposition can

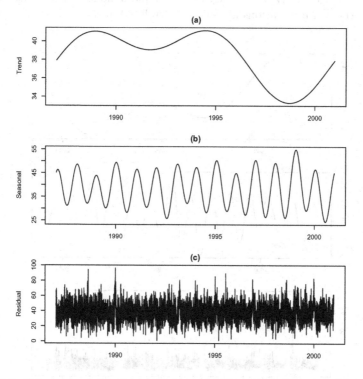

Fig. 5.7. Chicago mortality timescale decomposition, 1987–2000, into (a) long-term trend, (b) seasonality, and (c) short-term variation.

be conducted for the PM_{10} data, which we do below.

```
> pm10 <- with(data, pm10tmean + pm10mtrend)
> poll.dc <- tsdecomp(pm10, c(1, 2, 15,
+      5114))
```

Figure 5.8 shows the three timescales for the Chicago PM_{10} data in the same format as Figure 5.7.

```
> par(mfrow = c(3, 1), mar = c(3, 4, 1,
+      2) + 0.1)
> x <- seq(as.Date("1987-01-01"), as.Date("2000-12-31"),
+      "day")
```

```
> plot(x, poll.dc[, 1], type = "l", ylab = "Trend")
> plot(x, poll.dc[, 2], type = "l", ylab = "Seasonal")
> plot(x, poll.dc[, 3], type = "l", ylab = "Residual")
```

Comparing Figures 5.8 and 5.7 visually, we can see that the seasonal components of mortality and PM_{10} do not correspond and in fact appear negatively correlated. The long-term trend components seem to behave similarly in that they are both generally decreasing. From the plots alone, it is difficult to tell if the short-term fluctuations are in fact correlated at all.

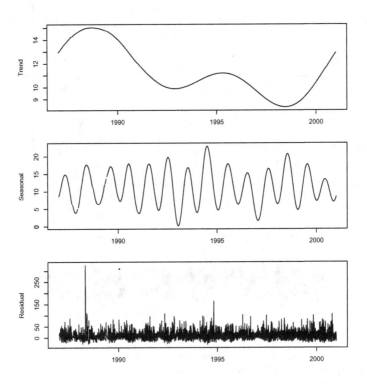

Fig. 5.8. Chicago PM_{10} timescale decomposition, 1987–2000

We can examine the correlations at different timescales more formally by actually computing the correlations separately for each timescale.

```
> c1 <- cor(mort.dc[, 1], poll.dc[, 1],
+     use = "complete.obs")
> c2 <- cor(mort.dc[, 2], poll.dc[, 2],
+     use = "complete.obs")
> c3 <- cor(mort.dc[, 3], poll.dc[, 3],
+     use = "complete.obs")
```

Doing so gives us a correlation of 0.65, for the long-term trend component
−0.81 for the seasonal component, and 0.12 for the short-term component.
Hence, the long-term and short-term timescales are positively correlated and
the seasonal timescale has a negative correlation. We had already suspected
the positive correlation in the long-term trends and the negative correlation
in the seasonality, but the positive correlation in the short-term variation is
interesting. Table 5.5 shows the correlations between mortality and PM_{10} for
each timescale in the context of Table 5.2.

	Trend	Mortality Seasonal	Short-Term
Trend	0.65		
Pollution Seasonal		-0.81	
Short-Term			0.12

Table 5.5. Correlations for mortality and PM_{10} at different timescales

An alternative and perhaps more flexible approach is to use linear regression to analyze everything at once and simultaneously conduct tests of
significance (if such tests are of interest).

```
> library(stats)
> poll.df <- as.data.frame(poll.dc)
> names(poll.df) <- c("Trend", "Season",
+      "ShortTerm")
> fit <- lm(death ~ Trend + Season + ShortTerm,
+      data = poll.df)
```

Table 5.6 shows the results of such a regression analysis. Because of the linear
model assumption and the orthogonality of the predictors, the results of the
regression analysis lead us to the same conclusions as the simple correlation
analysis.

	Estimate	Std. Error	t value	Pr(>|t|)
(Intercept)	118.5628	1.1507	103.04	0.0000
Trend	0.8299	0.0936	8.87	0.0000
Season	−1.2029	0.0375	−32.11	0.0000
ShortTerm	0.0714	0.0099	7.23	0.0000

Table 5.6. Regression of daily mortality on different timescales of PM_{10}

5.3.4 Looking at more detailed timescales

Although the long-term, seasonal, and short-term trends are common timescales
to examine in time series analysis, particular applications may allow for other

interesting and relevant timescales to examine. For example, in pollution studies one might be interested in separating out the effects of daily variation in
pollutant levels on mortality counts from the effects of weekly or monthly
variation.

The `tsdecomp` function can be used to look at more detailed timescales
of either pollution or mortality.

```
> freq.cuts <- c(1, 2, 15, round(5114/c(60,
+     30, 14, 7, 3.5)), 5114)
> poll.dc <- tsdecomp(pm10, freq.cuts)
> colnames(poll.dc) <- c("Long-term", "Seasonal",
+     "2-12 months", "1-2 months", "2-4 weeks",
+     "1-2 weeks", "3.5 days to 1 week",
+     "Less than 3.5 days")
```

We plot these more detailed timescales in Figure 5.9.

```
> par(mfcol = c(4, 2), mar = c(2, 2, 2,
+     2))
> x <- seq(as.Date("1987-01-01"), as.Date("2000-12-31"),
+     "day")
> cn <- colnames(poll.dc)
> for (i in 1:8) {
+     plot(x, poll.dc[, i], type = "l",
+         frame.plot = FALSE, main = cn[i],
+         ylab = "")
+ }
```

When looking at multiple timescales, it is a little easier to simply conduct
a multiple regression analysis of the outcome versus the timescales of the
pollutant rather than compute individual correlations.

```
> poll.df <- as.data.frame(poll.dc[, 1:8])
> fit <- lm(death ~ ., data = poll.df)
```

Table 5.7 shows the results of regressing all-cause nonaccidental mortality on
the eight timescales shown in Figure 5.9. Notice that the coefficients for the
"Long-term" and "Seasonal" timescales are identical to those in Table 5.6.
This is to be expected because of the linearity assumption and the orthogonality of the different timescales. However, now the short-term timescale has
been broken down even further so that we have estimates of the association
between mortality and timescales ranging from 2–12 months down to <3.5
days. Not all of the timescales could be considered statistically significant with
respect to their relationship with mortality. The summary in Table 5.6 provides a "breakdown" of the evidence for Chicago and allows for a potentially
more informed discussion of what evidence might be relevant for subsequent
decisions or actions.

Unfortunately, the timescale analysis using `tsdecomp()` can only be done
with cities that have relatively complete data on PM_{10}. In the next chapter

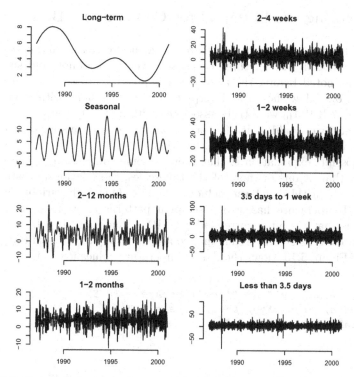

Fig. 5.9. Detailed timescale decomposition for Chicago, Illinois PM$_{10}$ data, 1987–2000.

	Estimate	Std. Error	t value	Pr($>|t|$)
(Intercept)	115.1945	0.5491	209.80	0.0000
Long-term	0.8300	0.0935	8.88	0.0000
Seasonal	−1.2029	0.0374	−32.15	0.0000
2-12 months	−0.0267	0.0363	−0.74	0.4623
1-2 months	0.0670	0.0421	1.59	0.1116
2-4 weeks	0.1251	0.0256	4.90	0.0000
1-2 weeks	0.1040	0.0197	5.27	0.0000
3.5 days to 1 week	0.0638	0.0184	3.46	0.0005
Less than 3.5 days	0.0364	0.0229	1.59	0.1121

Table 5.7. Regression of daily mortality on more detailed timescales of PM$_{10}$, Chicago, Illinois, 1987–2000

we use other methods to get around this limitation.

5.4 Exploring the Potential for Confounding Bias

Under the linear regression model, there is evidence of an association between mortality and PM_{10} at all three timescales (yearly, seasonal, and shorter). However, as noted before, the association is positive in two timescales and negative in one. How should we interpret these results along with the regression analysis? If PM_{10} were truly associated with mortality (either positively or negatively) we would at least expect that the correlations for each of the timescales would all be in the same direction.

One possible explanation is that there is some confounding going on. It is possible that at one or more of the timescales, the relationship is in fact confounded by a third not-yet-included variable. One such variable is temperature. Temperature has strong seasonal patterns as well as short-term fluctuations that are often correlated with PM_{10} and mortality. In addition, temperature has long-term trends that could potentially affect both PM_{10} and mortality. Figure 5.10 shows the daily temperature values for Chicago.

```
> data <- readCity("chic", collapseAge = TRUE)
> with(data, plot(date, tmpd, type = "l",
+      ylab = "Temperature"))
```

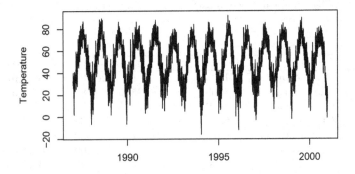

Fig. 5.10. Daily temperature for Chicago, 1987–2000.

We can remove the effect of temperature by regressing both mortality and PM_{10} on temperature and taking the residuals.

```
> temp <- data[, "tmpd"]
> pm10.r <- resid(lm(pm10 ~ temp, na.action = na.exclude))
> death.r <- resid(lm(death ~ temp, na.action = na.exclude))
```

```
> poll.dc <- tsdecomp(pm10.r, c(1, 2, 15,
+     5114))
```

Figure 5.11 shows a timescale decomposition of PM_{10} after the variation due to temperature has been removed.

```
> par(mfrow = c(3, 1), mar = c(3, 4, 1,
+     2) + 0.1)
> x <- seq(as.Date("1987-01-01"), as.Date("2000-12-31"),
+     "day")
> plot(x, poll.dc[, 1], type = "l", ylab = "Trend")
> plot(x, poll.dc[, 2], type = "l", ylab = "Seasonal")
> plot(x, poll.dc[, 3], type = "l", ylab = "Residual")
```

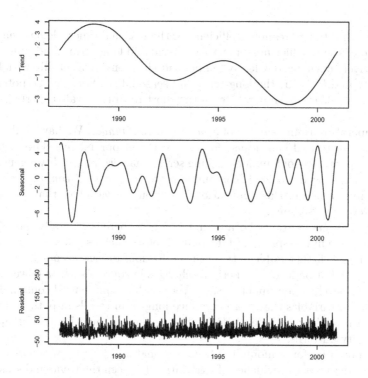

Fig. 5.11. Timescale decomposition of the residuals of PM_{10} regressed on temperature.

We can then take the mortality residuals and regress them on the timescale decomposition of the PM_{10} residuals.

```
> poll.df <- as.data.frame(poll.dc)
> names(poll.df) <- c("Trend", "Season",
+     "ShortTerm")
```

```
> fit <- lm(death.r ~ Trend + Season + ShortTerm,
+       data = poll.df)
```

Table 5.8 shows the estimated regression coefficients for the relationship between PM_{10} and mortality after removing temperature. Notice now in

	Estimate	Std. Error	t value	$Pr(>|t|)$
(Intercept)	−0.0988	0.1835	−0.54	0.5902
Trend	0.8829	0.0894	9.88	0.0000
Season	0.3226	0.0661	4.88	0.0000
ShortTerm	0.1061	0.0103	10.29	0.0000

Table 5.8. Regression of mortality on PM_{10} with temperature removed

Table 5.8 that the regression coefficient for the seasonal timescale has changed sign whereas the coefficients for the short-term and long-term trend timescales are relatively unchanged. Clearly temperature has some relationship with both mortality and PM_{10} at the long-term and seasonal timescales. The potential confounding effect of temperature on the short-term timescale is perhaps less substantial.

Temperature is an example of a *measured confounder*. We have daily data on temperature and can adjust for it directly in our models. Often, there are other potential confounders in time series analysis for which we generally do not have any data. Such confounders are *unmeasured confounders* and an example of one in this application is a group of variables that we might collectively call "season".

Season affects mortality because in the winter there is generally thought to be an increase in the spread of infectious diseases such as influenza. Unfortunately, there is little reliable data on such infectious disease events. Season can also affect pollution levels via periodic changes in sources such as power plant production levels or automobile usage. Yet another unmeasured confounder is the group of variables that might produce long-term trends in both pollution and mortality. As mentioned before, these include population demographics and activity patterns.

The potential for confounding from seasonal and long-term trends might lead us to discount the evidence of association between the trend and seasonal components found in Tables 5.5 and 5.6. In subsequent analyses we may wish to completely remove their influence on any assocations we choose to estimate.

We can observe the potential confounding effect of season on the relationship between PM_{10} and mortality by conducting a simple stratified analysis. We demonstrate this effect using data from New York City, New York.

```
> data <- readCity("ny", collapseAge = TRUE)
```

We can make a simple scatterplot of the daily mortality and PM_{10} data for the years 1987–2000.

```
> with(data, plot(l1pm10tmean, death,
                     xlab = expression(PM[10]),
+      ylab = "Daily mortality", cex = 0.6,
+      col = gray(0.4)))
```

We can also overlay a simple linear regression line on the plot to highlight the relationship between the two variables.

```
> f <- lm(death ~ l1pm10tmean, data)
> with(data, {
+      lines(sort(l1pm10tmean), predict(f,
+          data.frame(l1pm10tmean = sort(l1pm10tmean))),
+          lwd = 4)
+ })
```

The resulting scatterplot is shown in Figure 5.12. The PM_{10} data we have

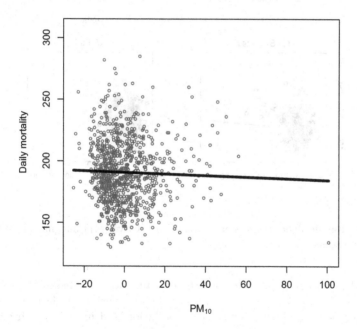

Fig. 5.12. Scatterplot of daily mortality and lag 1 PM_{10} for New York City, New York, 1987–2000.

chosen to plot is the lag 1 PM_{10} value. This means that for each day's mortality count, we plot the previous day's PM_{10} value. Time series studies of mortality and PM_{10} have shown this to be an important lag structure [101]. The overall relationship between lag 1 PM_{10} and mortality in New York City appears to be negative.

In Figures 5.13(a–d) we have plotted the New York City mortality and PM_{10} data four times, with each plot highlighting a different season of the year. Within each plot we have overlaid in black the data points corresponding to that season as well as the regression line fit to only the data from that season. We can see that for each season, the relationship between lag 1

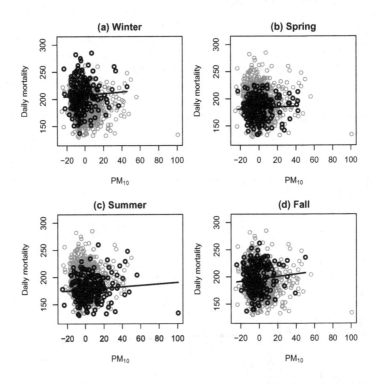

Fig. 5.13. Simple linear regression of New York City PM_{10} and mortality data, stratified by season.

PM_{10} and mortality is positive, but the overall, the relationship is negative, as shown in Figure 5.12. This example with New York City data illustrates how estimated associations between air pollution and mortality can change depending on whether one decides to adjust for season.

In general, without data on the factors that cause the seasonal and long-term trends we cannot adjust for them directly when modeling air pollution and mortality. However, one approach is to make an assumption that these variables affect mortality and pollution in a smooth manner. Given this assumption we can use a smooth function of time itself to adjust for the various seasonal and long-term trends that may confound the relationship between air pollution and mortality. We explore this approach to adjusting for unmeasured confounding in Chapter 6.

5.5 Summary

Many standard tools of statistical analysis can be brought to bear when analyzing time series data. Looking at correlations or simple linear regression models can provide insight into relationships between variables. In addition, smoothing techniques can be used for exploratory analysis.

With time series data, a feature that we can take advantage of is the fact that there is an underlying process evolving over time. We can meaningfully decompose a time series into a long-term trend, a seasonal pattern, and residual short-term variation. This kind of timescale decomposition can give us insight into where the evidence of an association exists. In epidemiological studies, there is an added benefit of timescale decompositions in that we can examine each timescale independently and evaluate the strength of the evidence.

For example, with air pollution and mortality, even though the associations at the long-term trend and seasonal timescales may be confounded, the variation at the short-term timescale is not necessarily confounded by the same factors and the associations there may still be credible. This fact highlights the benefits of the timescale decomposition. By decomposing the predictor into separate long-term trend, seasonal, and short-term timescales, we can isolate the sources of evidence and use our subject matter knowledge to upweight or downweight the evidence appropriately.

In any epidemiological study one might reasonably ask, "From where does the evidence of association come?" In air pollution and health time series studies it would appear that perhaps the most reliable evidence comes from the short-term timescale variation. We explore this question in greater depth in the chapters to follow.

5.6 Reproducibility Package

For the sake of brevity, some of the code for producing the analyses in this chapter has not been shown for the sake of brevity. However, the full data and code for reproducing all of the analyses and plots can be downloaded using the **cacher** package by calling

```
> clonecache(id = "2a04c4d5523816f531f98b141c0eb17c6273f308")
```

which will download the cached analysis from the Reproducible Research Archive.

5.7 Problems

In this set of problems we explore the daily time series data of air pollution and mortality and we visually inspect their long-term, seasonal, and short-term variation. We also calculate the associations between air pollution and mortality at these different scales of variation.

The data frames for each of the cities all have the same variable names. The primary variables we need from each data frame are

- `death`, daily mortality counts from all-cause non-accidental mortality
- `pm10tmean`, daily detrended, PM_{10} values
- `pm10mtrend`, daily median trend of PM_{10}
- `date`, the date, stored as an object of class `Date`
- `tmpd`, daily temperature

The data for a given city (denoted by its abbreviated name) can be read into R using the `readCity` function from the **NMMAPSlite** package described in Chapter 2.

1. Load data for Chicago (`chic`), New York (`ny`), and Los Angeles (`la`) into R.
2. For each city, plot the PM_{10} data versus date. Try plotting PM_{10} both with and without the trend added in. Try plotting the data in smaller windows of time to see more detail.
3. Using the `tsdecomp` function, decompose the Chicago PM_{10} data into three timescales: long-term variation, seasonal variation short-term variation. Plot your results.
4. For each of the three cities, plot the all-cause non-accidental mortality data versus date separately for each of the three age categories: `under65`, `65to74`, and `75p`.
5. Using the `tsdecomp` function, decompose the mortality data into three timescales (as before).
6. Revisit the timescale decompositions for both PM_{10} and mortality in Chicago. Visually compare the long-term trend for mortality with the long-term trend for PM_{10}. Do the same comparison for the seasonal and short-term components.
7. Compute the correlation coefficient between the long-term trends for mortality and PM_{10}. Compute the correlation coefficients for both the seasonal and short-term components of mortality and PM_{10}. If there are any missing data, set `use = "complete"` in the call to `cor` when computing the correlation.
8. Try the same timescale/correlation analysis with the city of Seattle, WA (`seat`). Do you get the same correlations?
9. Try the same timescale/correlation analysis with Pittsburgh, PA (`pitt`).
10. Fill in the following table with the correlations between PM_{10} and mortality computed at different timescales in the previous steps:

Long-Term	Seasonal	Short-Term
Chicago		
Seattle		
Pittsburgh		

Upon completing the problems above, consider the following questions.

1. What are the main characteristics of the time series data for mortality and air pollution?
2. What are the long-term, seasonal, and short-term variations in air pollution in U.S. cities? Are there differences between cities?
3. What are the long-term, seasonal, and short-term variations in mortality in U.S. cities? Are there differences between cities? Are there differences between age categories?
4. How do the long-term, seasonal, and short-term variations in PM_{10} and mortality relate to each other? How do they relate on different timescales?
5. Is there any evidence of an association between PM_{10} and mortality in these cities? Which timescale is more suitable for drawing inferences?
6. How should we weigh the evidence from the different timescales? What evidence is more important? What evidence should be discounted and why?

6

Statistical Models

6.1 Introduction

In this chapter we cover the array of statistical methods that are now in widespread use in air pollution and health research. The previous chapter focused on methods for exploring air pollution and health data and for examining general trends and associations. This chapter focuses on methods and models for obtaining risk estimates from time series data and exploring the sensitivity of those estimates to modeling approaches.

In addition to the **NMMAPSlite** package and its dependencies, you need the following packages for the examples in this chapter.

- **gam**, for generalized additive modeling capabilities, available on CRAN
- **tsModel**, for various time series modeling support functions

6.2 Models for Air Pollution and Health

In time series studies of air pollution and health, we typically model the outcome as a time series of counts representing the number of times a particular event has occurred on a given day. Each observation of the outcome Y_t could be a count indicating the number of deaths that occurred on day t or the number of hospitalizations for heart failure on day t. At the most basic level, we are trying to model the relationship between outcome Y and exposure X in the presence of potential confounding factors Z.

With time series of counts, the most commonly used model is the log-linear Poisson model. This model takes the outcome Y_t to be Poisson with mean μ_t and the log of μ_t is the linear predictor. The linear predictor typically includes terms for the exposure of interest (e.g., air pollution levels) and various potential confounders. Models often fall into the form

$$Y_t \quad \sim \text{Poisson}(\mu_t)$$
$$\log \mu_t = \alpha + \beta\, x_{t-\ell}$$
$$+ \boldsymbol{\eta}\, \text{measured confounders}_t \qquad (6.1)$$
$$+ \text{unmeasured confounders}_t$$

where the pollutant $x_{t-\ell}$ might be included in the model at a lag ℓ that might range from 0 for no lag to 13 for a two-week lag. Obviously, "unmeasured confounders" cannot be included directly in the model but here we take "unmeasured confounders" to mean a suitable proxy for any such variables. We discuss possible proxies later in this chapter.

In general for a time series model such as in (6.1), the target of inference is the effect of a unit increase in the exposure on a single day. The parameter β is the log-relative risk for $x_{t-\ell}$ and $100 \times (e^\beta - 1)$ measures the percent increase in mortality per unit increase in the pollutant. Other elements of the model, as indicated by their labels in (6.1), are factors that might confound the relationship between pollutant exposure and the outcome of interest.

In air pollution and health applications, the challenge is to obtain a good estimate of β in the presence of much more powerful signals. For example, factors such as temperature and season almost always have a strong relationship with mortality and so one must take care to remove the potential confounding effects of these factors. Furthermore, various factors for which no measurements are available can also confound the relationship between pollution and health so we must also gauge the sensitivity of estimates of β to potential unmeasured confounding.

Figure 6.1 illustrates the difficulty with estimating the effect of air pollution on health. Figure 6.1 is simply a plot of the fitted linear predictors for season, temperature, and PM_{10} when put in a model to predict daily nonaccidental mortality in Chicago, IL.

```
> chic <- readCity("chic", collapseAge = TRUE)
> fit <- glm(death ~ l1pm10tmean + ns(date,
+      4 * 14) + ns(tmpd, 6) + dow, data = chic,
+      na.action = na.exclude, family = poisson)
> pr <- predict(fit, type = "terms")
```

We can see clearly that season and temperature are very strong predictors of mortality whereas the PM_{10} signal is practically buried among the others. Extracting this PM_{10} signal is the key to time series modeling of air pollution and health.

In time series analyses of air pollution and health we must be careful to control for potential confounding from other time-varying predictors. Factors that vary across individuals or communities but do not vary substantially from day to day cannot confound the relationship between daily variation in air pollution and daily variation in health outcomes.

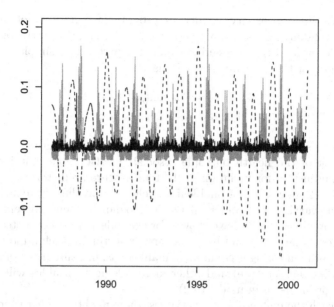

Fig. 6.1. Linear predictors for season/trend (dashed), temperature (solid gray), and PM$_{10}$ (solid black) for nonaccidental mortality in Chicago, IL, 1987–2000.

6.3 Semiparametric Models

Given the conceptual model in (6.1) which has an outcome, an exposure of interest, measured confounders, and potential unmeasured confounders, an attractive methodologic framework within which to work is one of *semiparametric models* [95]. Semiparametric models combine the advantages of parametric and nonparametric models by allowing for the inclusion of explicit parametric terms for certain predictors (such as an exposure of interest) and smooth nonparametric terms for other predictors.

The specific type of semiparametric model that we use is a *generalized additive model* (GAM) where log μ_t is assumed to be additive in its predictors but not necessarily linear [45]. GAMs provide some flexibility for using nonlinear or nonparametric terms but do not suffer from the curse of dimensionality as do other more flexible nonparametric methods such as kernel smoothing or local polynomial modeling. Although the additivity assumption is strong, GAMs still provide a very flexible framework for modeling and exploratory analysis. The use of GAMs in air pollution and health was proposed in [106] and has since become a standard method in this area.

Suppose in a given city, county, or geographic region, we observe y_t, a time series of daily mortality counts $(t = 1, \ldots, n)$, x_t a time series of daily air pollution levels, and z_t a time series of daily temperature. A simple generalized linear model for the outcome y_t would have

$$Y_t \sim \text{Poisson}(\mu_t)$$
$$\log \mu_t = \alpha + \beta\, x_{t-\ell} + \eta\, z_t \qquad (6.2)$$

Again, in this model we are primarily interested in estimating β, the log-relative risk of the health outcome associated with a one unit increase in pollution, adjusting for variation in the temperature predictor z_t.

Model (6.2) might be reasonable if we believed that there were no other potential time-varying confounders in addition to daily current day temperature. However, previous studies have shown, for example, that other meteorological factors such as humidity can be important predictors in such a model. Given that weather monitoring is common in many areas, measurements of humidity (or dewpoint temperature) and other meteorological variables will likely be available for inclusion in model (6.2).

Even with the meteorological variables, there might be other time-varying factors for which we do not have daily measurements that could confound the relationship between x_t and y_t. At a minimum, it would be an incomplete analysis to estimate β without fully understanding the sensitivity of that estimate to other possible model formulations. Unfortunately, without direct measurements, we cannot include such potential confounders into model (6.2). However, we can make an assumption that these other factors vary smoothly with time. We may not be able to specify exactly how they vary, however, we might assume that they are not too wiggly from day to day.

Given this assumption, we can use a smooth function of time itself to serve as a proxy for those unmeasured confounders, expanding model (6.2) to be

$$\log \mu_t = \alpha + \beta\, x_{t-\ell} + \eta\, z_t + s(t, \lambda) \qquad (6.3)$$

Here, $s(t, \lambda)$ is used to indicate a smooth function of time t. The smoothness of the function is controlled by a scalar parameter λ, also known as the *smoothing parameter* or *degrees of freedom*. In this setting, larger values of λ indicate a less smooth (rougher) function of time and smaller values indicate a smoother function.

In addition to including a smooth function of time, we may wish to allow for nonlinear relationships between the outcome and the measured predictors. For example, temperature is known to have a nonlinear relationship with mortality in some regions [17]. Such a nonlinear relationship reflects the fact that in the winter, increases in temperature can be beneficial and decrease mortality whereas in the summer, temperature increases can be harmful.

With GAMs we can allow for nonlinear relationships between measured predictors and the outcome by adjusting model (6.3) to be

$$\log \mu_t = \alpha + \beta\, x_{t-\ell} + s(z_t, \lambda_1) + s(t, \lambda_2) \qquad (6.4)$$

This model indicates that z_t (temperature) has a smooth but otherwise unspecified relationship with mortality. The smoothness is controlled by the degrees of freedom λ_1.

So far, we have provided a basic introduction to how the conceptual model in (6.1) can be implemented using semiparametric GAMs. In the subsequent sections we describe how to use various R packages to fit such models to air pollution and health data and how to interpret the results.

6.3.1 GAMs in R

The world of GAMs in R is varied and diverse with a number of different packages implementing different approaches. We list a few that are available as of version 2.7.0 of R.

- **mgcv:** This package is a "Recommended" package for R and should be present in every installation. It is written by Simon Wood and it implements GAMs as well as generalized additive mixed models (GAMMs) via penalized splines. Smoothing parameters can be estimated using generalized cross-validation (GCV) or unbiased risk estimation (UBRE).
- **gam:** Written by Trevor Hastie, this package provides functions originally available in S-PLUS and is available from CRAN. GAMs can be fit using loess or smoothing splines. There are no methods here for smoothing parameter estimation.
- **splines:** This package is a base package for R and contains a number of functions that can be used to fit flexible regression models. For example, the bs() and ns() functions can be used to set up B-spline or natural spline bases, respectively. Although these models are strictly speaking parametric, they still offer far more flexibility than purely linear alternatives. In addition, fully parameteric models can often be faster to fit with larger datasets.
- **mda:** This package is available from CRAN and contains the function bruto that can fit additive models via smoothing splines. However, because it is limited to fitting Gaussian regression models, it is ultimately not of much use to us here.

In this chapter we primarily use the **gam** and **splines** packages to fit generalized additive models. However, most of what we demonstrate here could also be implemented via the **mgcv** package.

6.4 Pollutants: The Exposure of Interest

Our ability to estimate the effect of air pollution on daily mortality will typically depend on the availability of the data. Pollutant data are measured according to a variety of sampling schemes, depending on the nature of the pollutant. Gaseous pollutants tend to be measured every day, although sometimes they are only measured during certain seasons. For example, ozone in the United States is often only measured during the months of April through September. Particulate matter (both PM_{10} and $PM_{2.5}$) is usually not measured every day but rather once every three days or once every six days.

6.4.1 Single versus distributed lag

In the model described in (6.1), an assumption is made that the effect of a unit increase only plays out over a single day, determined by the lag ℓ. A unit increase in pollution on day t is associated with a change in mortality ℓ days later. Model (6.1) is sometimes referred to as a single lag model because of this assumption. Identifying the appropriate lag of the exposure to include in the model is a problem that generally needs to be guided by subject matter knowledge. For example, with a mortality outcome, it is uncommon to see an association with a pollutant for more than a few days into the future. However, with hospitalizations or other morbidity outcomes, one can potentially observe an association extending to a week or more.

An alternative to single lag models is a *distributed lag model*, where multiple lags of pollution are included in the model simultaneously. Such a model typically has the form

$$\log \mu_t = \alpha + \sum_{\ell=0}^{K} \beta_\ell \, x_{t-\ell} + \text{other factors}_t \tag{6.5}$$

where K is the maximum lag. Values of K in the literature range from 2 days up to 40 days [e.g., 128, 6, 33]. Distributed lag models assume that the effect of a unit increase in pollution on a given day is spread out over K days into the future. Although such a model is arguably more realistic, there are a number of challenges to fitting distributed lag models that must be considered.

Single lag models, which assume that a unit increase in pollution affects mortality a fixed number of days in the future, can be fit as long as pollutant data are available. Distributed lag models can only be fit if pollutant data are available every day. Therefore, our ability to fit distributed lag models for particulate matter is greatly hindered by the sampling scheme for the pollutant.

As an example, we can fit single lag models to the Chicago, IL data and list the estimates of the PM_{10} coefficient by lag.

```
> data <- readCity("chic")
```

Here we fit a separate model for PM_{10} at lag 0, 1, 2, 3, and 4. Each of the models also includes an age category specific intercept and current day temperature.

```
> f0 <- glm(death ~ pm10tmean + tmpd + agecat,
+     data = data, family = poisson)
> f1 <- glm(death ~ Lag(pm10tmean, 1, agecat) +
+     tmpd + agecat, data = data, family = poisson)
> f2 <- glm(death ~ Lag(pm10tmean, 2, agecat) +
+     tmpd + agecat, data = data, family = poisson)
> f3 <- glm(death ~ Lag(pm10tmean, 3, agecat) +
+     tmpd + agecat, data = data, family = poisson)
> f4 <- glm(death ~ Lag(pm10tmean, 4, agecat) +
+     tmpd + agecat, data = data, family = poisson)
> ss <- list(summary(f0), summary(f1), summary(f2),
+     summary(f3), summary(f4))
> models <- lapply(ss, function(x) x$coefficients[2,
+     c("Estimate", "Std. Error")])
```

Table 6.1 shows the estimates of the PM_{10} coefficient from five different single lag models. The estimates for lags 0 and 1 are relatively close but the estimates

	Estimate	Std. Error
Lag 0 PM10	0.000931	0.000074
Lag 1 PM10	0.000728	0.000073
Lag 2 PM10	0.000164	0.000072
Lag 3 PM10	0.000077	0.000072
Lag 4 PM10	−0.000053	0.000072

Table 6.1. Results from single lag models, Chicago, IL, 1987–2000

for lags 2, 3, and 4 are much smaller (and even negative for lag 4).

Distributed lag models can often be fit to gaseous pollutant data such as ozone, which has already been done on a national scale [see e.g. 6]. In order to fit distributed lag models for particulate matter one must resort either to examining a small subset of cities with everyday PM measurements or filling in missing PM data via an imputation method. The former has been done in a few locations [e.g., 112], however, the latter is still an active research area.

Because Chicago, IL has everyday PM_{10} data, we can fit a distributed lag model to those data and compare the estimates of the lagged effects with those from single lag models.

```
> data <- readCity("chic")
> fit <- glm(death ~ Lag(pm10tmean, 0:4,
+     agecat) + tmpd + agecat, data = data,
+     family = poisson)
> summ <- summary(fit)
```

Table 6.2 shows the results from the distributed lag models. Generally, the estimates for the individual lags tell a similar story as in Table 6.1 in that the estimated coefficients for lag 0 and 1 are larger than those for lags 2–4. One

	Estimate	Std. Error	z value	$\Pr(>|z|)$
(Intercept)	3.607541	0.004984	723.88	0.00
Lag(pm10tmean, 0:4, agecat)0	0.000794	0.000084	9.46	0.00
Lag(pm10tmean, 0:4, agecat)1	0.000471	0.000090	5.23	0.00
Lag(pm10tmean, 0:4, agecat)2	−0.000051	0.000090	−0.56	0.57
Lag(pm10tmean, 0:4, agecat)3	0.000197	0.000090	2.20	0.03
Lag(pm10tmean, 0:4, agecat)4	−0.000062	0.000083	−0.74	0.46
tmpd	−0.003067	0.000085	−36.24	0.00
agecat65to74	−0.227776	0.004095	−55.63	0.00
agecat75p	0.607963	0.003388	179.43	0.00

Table 6.2. Results from distributed lag model, Chicago, IL, 1987–2000

anomaly is the sudden increase in the estimated coefficient for lag 3, which is bigger than the single lag estimate for lag 3.

Distributed lag models can be used to estimate the "total" or cumulative effect of an air pollution episode, which in the context of the log-linear model can be thought of as the cumulative percent increase in mortality associated with a unit increase in air pollution on a given day. For example, if we assume that a unit increase in air pollution on a given day only plays out over K days into the future, as in (6.5), and if we imagine that $x_0 = 1$, and $x_1 = x_2 = \cdots = 0$ (i.e. a spike at $t = 0$), then the cumulative effect of the unit increase at time $t = 0$ is

$$\text{Cumulative effect} = \gamma = \sum_{\ell=0}^{K} \beta_\ell$$

The interpretation of γ is similar to that of β in (6.1); that is, $100 \times (e^\gamma - 1)$ is the percent increase in mortality over $K + 1$ days associated with a 1 unit increase in pollution on a single day.

```
> rn <- rownames(summ$coefficients)
> i <- grep("pm10tmean", rn, fixed = TRUE)
> coefs <- summ$coefficients[i, "Estimate"]
> total <- sum(coefs)
```

It is not possible to tell beforehand whether the cumulative effect will be bigger or smaller than the single lag estimate. With more immediate relationships where most of the association is observed in early lags, the single lag estimates and cumulative effect estimates will usually be close. However, if the association plays out over many days, single lag estimates may be smaller. The estimate of the cumulative effect in the Chicago, IL distributed lag model in Table 6.2 is 0.00135, which can be interpreted as a 1.35 percent increase in mortality associated with a 10 $\mu g/m^3$ increase in PM_{10}. This effect is bigger than any of the estimates from the single lag models.

6.4.2 Mortality displacement

There is one scenario where distributed lag estimates of the cumulative effect may be smaller than estimates from single lag models. The "harvesting hypothesis" (also known as "mortality displacement") states that short-term increases in air pollution only affect a frail pool of individuals that are particularly susceptible [129, 109, 110, 128, 125, 32]. In the event of an increase in pollutant levels, these frail people are removed from the population at risk (either through death or hospitalization), leaving a depleted frail pool. Therefore, on subsequent days, we might observe lower than expected levels of the outcome. In such a scenario, the cumulative effect over a short time period might be zero because the higher than expected response close to the day of the increased exposure is balanced by the lower than expected response on subsequent days.

6.5 Modeling Measured Confounders

Measured confounders consist of predictors that vary from day to day in a manner similar to that of air pollution and mortality. These predictors have the potential to explain the covariation in pollution and mortality and might lead us to incorrectly attribute the observed effect to air pollution. With measured confounders, we have the data required to adjust for the variables directly in any statistical model, so that we can attempt to remove the variation attributable to the confounder before examining the relationship of interest.

One important measured variable is the "weather," which we can crudely break down into temperature and humidity (or dewpoint temperature). Both temperature and dewpoint temperature have well-known relationships to both air pollution and health [54, 97].

Temperature has an interesting relationship with mortality in that an increase in temperature can be harmful or beneficial depending on the time of the year. In summertime, short-term increases in temperature are generally associated with increases in mortality whereas in wintertime, short-term increases in temperature are associated with decreases in mortality [17]. Furthermore, mortality in summertime is related to increases in temperature on the order of 1–2 days. In wintertime, mortality is more closely related to long stretches of cold days in a row. Therefore, one may need to consider looking simultaneously at the current day temperature and the temperatures from previous days. Hence, we may need a distributed lag model for temperature to capture this phenomenon [123].

We can explore the confounding effect of temperature by including it directly in our log-linear Poisson model; that is,

$$\log \mu_t = \alpha + \beta\, x_{t-1} + \sum_{k=0}^{K} \eta_k\, z_{t-k} \tag{6.6}$$

where mortality Y_t is distributed as Poisson with mean μ_t, z_{t-k} is the temperature for day t at lag k, and x_{t-1} is lag 1 PM_{10}. We can vary the value of K, the maximum number of temperature lags, to see how the estimate of β changes as more temperature lags are included. We can illustrate this effect with data from New York City, New York.

```
> data.c <- readCity("ny", collapseAge = TRUE)
```

Using a range of temperature lags ranging from 0 to 13 days, we fit 14 different models and examine the resulting regression coefficient for the lag 1 PM_{10} variable.

```
> maxlag <- 0:13
> models <- sapply(maxlag, function(mlag) {
+       fit <- glm(death ~ l1pm10tmean + Lag(tmpd,
+           seq(0, mlag)), data = data.c,
+           family = poisson)
+       summ <- summary(fit)
+       summ.coef <- summ$coefficients["l1pm10tmean",
+           2]
+       c(coef(fit)["l1pm10tmean"], summ.coef)
+ })
```

Figure 6.2 shows the coefficient for lag 1 PM_{10} from a Poisson generalized linear model versus the number of lags of temperature included in the model (i.e. the value of K).

```
> rng <- range(models[1, ] - 1.96 * models[2,
+       ], models[1, ] + 1.96 * models[2,
+       ], 0)
> par(mar = c(4, 5, 1, 1))
> plot(maxlag, models[1, ], type = "b",
+       pch = 20, ylim = rng, xlab = "Maximum temperature lag",
+       ylab = expression(hat(beta) * " for " *
+           PM[10] * " at lag 1"))
> lines(maxlag, models[1, ] + 1.96 * models[2,
+       ], lty = 2)
> lines(maxlag, models[1, ] - 1.96 * models[2,
+       ], lty = 2)
> abline(h = 0, lty = 3)
```

For maximum lag 0, we only include the current day's temperature; for maximum lag 13 we include the previous two weeks' daily temperature values in the model. From Figure 6.2 we see that the estimate of the pollution effect $\hat{\beta}$ is strongly affected by the number of lags of temperature included in the model. In particular, the estimate of the PM_{10} coefficient drops by almost 50% between one and five lags of temperature.

However, recall that the effect of temperature on mortality can differ by season. One might think of temperature as having a "cold" relationship and a "warm" relationship with mortality. Given that, we might want to look

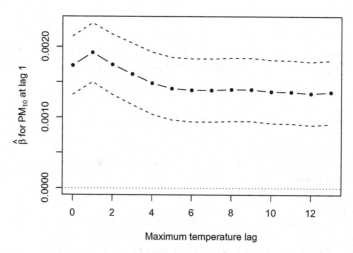

Fig. 6.2. Association between lag 1 PM_{10} and mortality ( ) as the number of lags of temperature included in the model is increased, New York, NY, 1987–2000.

separately at the warm season and the cold season. We can do this by directly subsetting the data by season. First we can estimate the model in the "warm" season (spring and summer),

```
> data <- readCity("ny", collapseAge = TRUE)
> maxlag <- 0:13
> data.warm <- subset(data, quarters(date) %in%
+     c("Q2", "Q3"))
> models.warm <- sapply(maxlag, function(mlag) {
+     fit <- glm(death ~ l1pm10tmean + Lag(tmpd,
+         seq(0, mlag)), data = data.warm,
+         family = poisson)
+     summ <- summary(fit)
+     summ.coef <- summ$coefficients["l1pm10tmean",
+         2]
+     c(coef(fit)["l1pm10tmean"], summ.coef)
+ })
```

and then we can fit the same models for the "cold" season (fall and winter).

```
> data.cold <- subset(data, quarters(date) %in%
+     c("Q1", "Q4"))
> models.cold <- sapply(maxlag, function(mlag) {
+     fit <- glm(death ~ l1pm10tmean + Lag(tmpd,
+         seq(0, mlag)), data = data.cold,
+         family = poisson)
+     summ <- summary(fit)
+     summ.coef <- summ$coefficients["l1pm10tmean",
+         2]
```

```
+        c(coef(fit)["l1pm10tmean"], summ.coef)
+ })
```

In Figure 6.3 we have created the same picture that is in Figure 6.2 except
we have created separate pictures for warm and cold seasons.

```
> trellis.par.set(theme = canonical.theme("pdf",
+       FALSE))
> y <- c(models.warm[1, ], models.cold[1,
+       ])
> xpts <- rep(maxlag, 2)
> f <- gl(2, length(maxlag), labels = c("Warm season",
+       "Cold season"))
> std <- c(models.warm[2, ], models.cold[2,
+       ])
> rng <- range(y - 1.96 * std, y + 1.96 *
+       std, 0)
> rng <- rng + c(-1, 1) * 0.05 * diff(rng)
> ylab <- expression(hat(beta) * " for " *
+       PM[10] * " at lag 1")
> p <- xyplot(y ~ xpts | f, as.table = TRUE,
+       ylim = rng, subscripts = TRUE, panel = function(x,
+           y, subscripts, ...) {
+           panel.xyplot(x, y, ...)
+           llines(x, y - 1.96 * std[subscripts],
+               lty = 2)
+           llines(x, y + 1.96 * std[subscripts],
+               lty = 2)
+           panel.abline(h = 0, lty = 3)
+       }, xlab = "Maximum temperature lag",
+       layout = c(1, 2), type = "b", ylab = ylab,
+       pch = 20)
> print(p)
```

The warm season is defined as April through September and the cold season
is defined as October through March. Figure 6.3 shows that for the warm
season, the number of lags of temperature included in the model does not
seem to be related to the estimate of the coefficient for lag 1 PM_{10}. However,
for the cold season, the estimate of the coefficient drops dramatically as the
number of lags of temperature included in the model increases from 1 to 5. For
both seasons, after including five lags of temperature, the association between
PM_{10} and mortality does not seem to change and is stable at approximately
the same value for both seasons. Here we can see that all of the variation
we observed in Figure 6.2 can be attributed to the variation in the estimate
during the cold season.

For New York City, the effect of PM_{10} on mortality during cold months
appears to be sensitive to the specification of temperature in the model. However, in model (6.6) we did not include any terms to control for the possible
seasonal factors that predict PM_{10} and mortality. When we modify model (6.6)

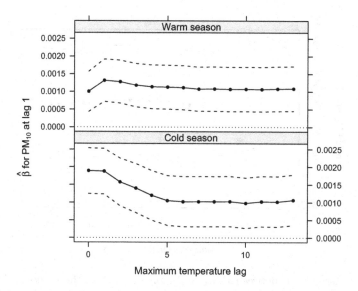

Fig. 6.3. Association between PM_{10} and mortality ( ) as the number of lags of temperature included in the model is increased, stratified by warm and cold seasons, New York City, 1987–2000.

to include a smooth function of time,

$$\log \mu_t = \alpha + \beta\, x_{t-1} + s(t, \lambda) + \sum_{k=0}^{K} \eta_k\, z_{t-k}$$

the results are different from Figure 6.2. Figure 6.4 shows the estimates of the PM_{10} coefficient as the maximum number of lags for temperature included in the model is increased for the model that includes a smooth function of time.

```
> data.c <- readCity("ny", collapseAge = TRUE)
> maxlag <- 0:13
> models <- sapply(maxlag, function(mlag) {
+     fit <- glm(death ~ l1pm10tmean + ns(date,
+         4 * 14) + Lag(tmpd, seq(0, mlag)),
+         data = data.c, family = poisson)
+     summ <- summary(fit)
+     summ.coef <- summ$coefficients["l1pm10tmean",
+         2]
+     c(coef(fit)["l1pm10tmean"], summ.coef)
+ })
```

Now we see that the the estimated coefficient is relatively stable across the entire range of lags.

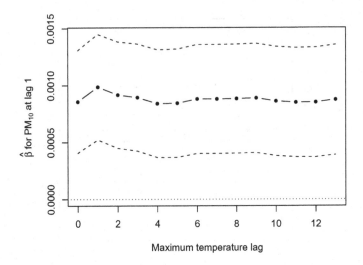

Fig. 6.4. Association between PM_{10} and mortality ( ) as the number of lags of temperature included in the model is increased, New York City, 1987–2000. Here the model includes a smooth function of time with four degrees of freedom per year to control for seasonal effects.

In [123] the authors looked extensively at the question of how temperature confounds the effect of PM_{10} on mortality. By using a vast array of distributed lag models with flexible specifications, they found that estimates are relatively insensitive to the choice of temperature model, as long as some minimal representation is included. Estimates from multisite studies were particularly robust to the specification of the temperature model.

6.6 Accounting for Unmeasured Confounders

In the previous chapter, we decomposed both the pollution series and the mortality series into three timescales: long-term trend, seasonal, and daily. One purpose of this decomposition was to identify timescales at which the relationship between the exposure and response were potentially least confounded by other time-varying predictors.

As mentioned in Section 6.3, one useful assumption to make about any potential unmeasured confounders is that they vary smoothly in time. With that assumption we can use a smooth function of time to adjust for those unmeasured confounders. In addition, the flexibility of using a smooth function allows us to gauge the sensitivity of our findings to various model specifications.

Using a smooth function of time to control for unmeasured confounders is similar in many ways to the timescale analysis that we conducted in the previous chapter. The inclusion of the smooth term in the model in a sense acts as a filter on the exposure and response and removes variation at a "timescale" determined by the degrees of freedom; our analysis is based on the residual variation in those variables. Using an arbitrary smooth function of time is a more flexible approach than using the Fourier basis in the timescale decomposition because we can choose to use a basis where each component is localized to a specific area as opposed to the global sine and cosine functions used in the Fourier basis.

With the smooth function of time the number of degrees of freedom specified will control the "timescale" at which we compare pollution levels with mortality counts. Small degrees of freedom, indicating a very smooth function, allow comparisons at longer timescales. Large degrees of freedom, indicating a very rough function, allow comparisons at much shorter timescales while setting aside any information at longer timescales. This approach can be thought of as regressing residuals from the smoothed dependent variable on residuals from the smoothed regressors. The smooth function of time serves as a linear filter on the mortality and pollution series and can remove any seasonal or long-term trends in the data.

The inclusion of a smooth function of time in a regression model introduces important statistical issues. One generally does not know precisely the complexity of the seasonal and long-term trends in the mortality time series or in the pollution time series. Therefore, a controversial issue is determining how much smoothness one should allow for the smooth function of time. This decision is critical because it determines the amount of residual temporal variation in mortality available to estimate the air pollution effect. Over-smoothing the series (thereby under-smoothing the residuals) can leave temporal cycles in the residuals that can produce confounding bias; under-smoothing the series (thereby over-smoothing the residuals) can remove too much temporal variability and potentially attenuate a true pollution effect. The decision is analogous to the situation in the previous chapter where we had to choose which timescales we thought would provide the most reliable evidence (i.e., least confounded). Current approaches to choosing the amount of smoothness include automatic, data-driven methods that choose the degree of smoothness by minimizing a goodness-of-fit criterion and methods based on prior knowledge of the timescales where confounding is more likely to occur.

To summarize, when including a smooth function of time in a time series model to adjust for potential smoothly varying confounders, the primary statistical questions of interest are:

1. How should the smooth function of time be represented?
2. Exactly how smooth should this smooth function be?

A number of approaches to representing the smooth functions have been used in the literature including smoothing splines, penalized splines, and parametric (natural) splines [31, 91, 112, 120, 46]. Other possibilities include using loess or kernel smoothers [106].

6.6.1 Using GAMs for air pollution and health

In this section we demonstrate how GAMs can be used to control for smoothly varying unmeasured confounders in time series models of air pollution and health. We make use of the **gam** and **splines** packages in our code examples.

To begin with we use the Denver, Colorado data to demonstrate the various methods. This dataset can be loaded from the **NMMAPSlite** package.

```
> data.raw <- readCity("denv", collapseAge = TRUE)
```

We can use the gam function from the **gam** package to first smooth the mortality and PM_{10} data and see the affects of using different degrees of freedom for the smooth function of time. Figure 6.5 shows the Denver nonaccidental mortality data (all ages) with two smoothers overlaid, one using 2 degrees of freedom per year of data and one using 12 degrees of freedom per year of data. Here we fit the simple model

$$Y_t \sim \text{Poisson}(\mu_t)$$
$$\log \mu_t = \alpha + s(t, df \times \ \# \text{ years of data})$$

where df is 2 or 12.

```
> xpts <- seq(as.Date("1987-01-01"), as.Date("2000-12-31"),
+     "day")
> fit2 <- gam(death ~ s(date, 2 * 14), family = poisson,
+     data = data.raw)
> p2 <- predict(fit2, data.frame(date = xpts),
+     type = "response")
> fit12 <- gam(death ~ s(date, 12 * 14),
+     family = poisson, data = data.raw)
> p12 <- predict(fit12, data.frame(date = xpts),
+     type = "response")
```

Because there are 14 years of data in the dataset this amounts to using 28 and 168 total degrees of freedom in the smoother. We have chosen to use smoothing splines in this particular example.

The 2 degree of freedom (per year) smoother clearly highlights the long-term increase in mortality in Denver, most likely due to a corresponding increase in population. Also, the seasonal pattern of mortality is clear, with winter peaks and summer troughs. The 12 degree of freedom (per year) smoother shows some of the more short-term fluctuations in the data and also more accurately captures the sharp peaks and troughs in the data.

A general principle that applies to nonparametric smoothers is the bias-variance trade-off with respect to the number of degrees of freedom allowed in the smoother. Smoothers with small degrees of freedom have difficulty capturing sharp increases or decreases and are more biased in those areas. With more degrees of freedom and flexibility, one can reduce the bias in those areas. However, with fewer degrees of freedom, a smoother is typically less flexible than a smoother with many degrees of freedom.

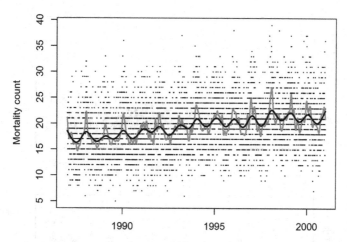

Fig. 6.5. Smooth of nonaccidental mortality for all ages using smoothing splines with 2 (black) and 12 (gray) degrees of freedom per year as the smoothing parameter, Denver, Colorado, 1987–2000.

Figure 6.6 shows the PM_{10} and ozone data for Denver with both 2 and 12 degree of freedom smoothing splines overlaid. We first fit a GAM to the PM_{10} data as a function of time

```
> xpts <- seq(as.Date("1987-01-01"), as.Date("2000-12-31"),
+     "day")
> fit2pm10 <- gam(pm10tmean ~ s(date, 2 *
+     14), data = data.raw)
> p2pm10 <- predict(fit2pm10, data.frame(date = xpts))
> fit12pm10 <- gam(pm10tmean ~ s(date, 12 *
+     14), data = data.raw)
> p12pm10 <- predict(fit12pm10, data.frame(date = xpts))
```

and then to the ozone data.

```
> xpts <- seq(as.Date("1987-01-01"), as.Date("2000-12-31"),
+     "day")
> fit2o3 <- gam(o3tmean ~ s(date, 2 * 14),
+     data = data.raw)
> p2o3 <- predict(fit2o3, data.frame(date = xpts))
> fit12o3 <- gam(o3tmean ~ s(date, 12 *
+     14), data = data.raw)
> p12o3 <- predict(fit12o3, data.frame(date = xpts))
```

A similar pattern is observed with these data as with the mortality data. One feature of interest is the much more obvious seasonal pattern in the ozone data. Ozone is a pollutant that depends critically on atmospheric conditions for its formation and is therefore more tightly correlated with seasonal patterns.

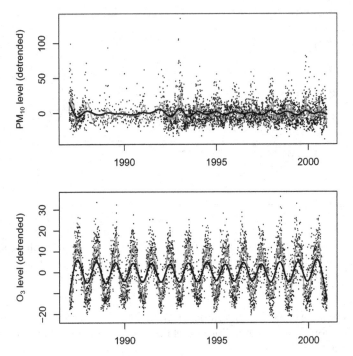

Fig. 6.6. Smooth of (detrended) PM_{10} and ozone using smoothing splines with 2 (black) and 12 (gray) degrees of freedom per year as the smoothing parameter, Denver, Colorado, 1987–2000.

Along with bias–variance considerations, in time series applications, one must also determine which timescale one is interested in to study the pollutant–mortality relationship. The number of degrees of freedom used in the smoother for time will determine the nature of the variation left over to estimate the risk from air pollution.

Our simple model incorporating both mortality and pollution is

$$Y_t \sim \text{Poisson}(\mu_t)$$
$$\log \mu_t = \alpha + \beta \, x_t + \eta \, z_t + s(t, df) \tag{6.7}$$

where Y_t is the mortality count, x_t is our pollutant predictor, z_t is temperature, and df is understood to mean $df \times$ # years of data. The target of inference is β and our goal is to estimate it while simultaneously controlling for measured and unmeasured confounders. We do not include a distributed lag for temperature here as in model (6.6) because Figure 6.4 indicated that the estimate of β is not affected much by the inclusion of other temperature lags once a smooth function of time is included in the model.

To see the effect of varying the degrees of freedom used in the smooth function of time, we can fit the model in (6.7) repeatedly, each time with a different smoothing parameter. Here we repeatedly fit a model nonaccidental mortality versus lag 1 PM_{10}, temperature, and a smooth function of time.

```
> dfValues <- c(2, 4, 6, 8, 10, 12, 14)
> control <- gam.control(epsilon = 0.00000001,
+      bf.epsilon = 0.00000001)
> modelsGAM <- sapply(dfValues, function(dfVal) {
+      total.df <- dfVal * 14
+      fit <- gam(death ~ l1pm10tmean + tmpd +
+          s(date, total.df), data = data.raw,
+          family = poisson, control = control)
+      gamex <- gam.exact(fit)
+      gamex.coef <- gamex$coefficients["l1pm10tmean",
+          "A-exact SE"]
+      c(coef(fit)["l1pm10tmean"], gamex.coef)
+ })
```

Figure 6.7(a) shows the different values of the PM_{10} coefficients that are estimated for each degrees of freedom. One can see that there is almost a two-fold range in the estimates of the log-relative risk, with the largest estimate associated with 2 df per year and the smallest estimate associated with 8 df per year.

From Figures 6.5 and 6.6 we know that at 2 df per year, only the long-term trend and seasonality are removed from both the PM_{10} and mortality series. Other subseasonal and shorter-term variations remain in the data. At 12 or 14 df per year, all variation in mortality and PM_{10} longer than about a one week timescale is removed and the log-relative risk is estimated by examining residual fluctuations on a subweek timescale.

The large estimate at 2 df per year in Figure 6.7 indicates that there is a 1.11 percent increase in mortality for a 10 $\mu g/m^3$ increase in PM_{10}. Although this estimate is intriguing, we may choose to discount it because it is more likely confounded by factors that can covary with mortality and PM_{10} at the subseasonal timescale.

As more variation in mortality and PM_{10} is removed in the 10–14 df per year range, the log-relative risk estimates appear to change little. There is certainly the potential for confounding in this range, but one could argue that there are fewer factors that might covary with both mortality and PM_{10} at the subweek/daily timescale. The estimates in this range, one might argue, are more reliable and less confounded.

The purpose of this analysis is not to conclusively identify the "correct" amount of smoothing to use, that is, the "right" number of degrees of freedom, but to show what the data say about the relationship between PM_{10} and mortality and to show from where the evidence of association comes. As in the previous chapter, we might feel more confident with estimates obtained from looking at shorter timescales than those obtained from looking at longer-term trends. However, the decision of what evidence to believe and what evidence to discount is one that can be made in conjunction with scientific expertise.

6.6.2 Computing standard errors for parametric terms in GAMs

In [31] the authors showed that the default method used by gam for estimating the standard error of the coefficient of a parametric term can be incorrect in the presence of strong concurvity. The **gam** package has a function gam.exact which implements the methods of [28] to calculate asymptotically exact standard errors from a gam model fit. The function can be applied to a "gam" object after the model has been fit. We used the gam.exact function for producing the approximate standard errors and confidence intervals shown in Figure 6.7.

An alternative approach is to use a fully parametric model via natural splines. With a fully parametric model, one can use standard methods for obtaining standard errors and approximate confidence intervals.

```
> dfValues <- c(2, 4, 6, 8, 10, 12, 14)
> modelsGLM <- sapply(dfValues, function(dfVal) {
+       total.df <- dfVal * 14
+       fit <- glm(death ~ l1pm10tmean + tmpd +
+           ns(date, total.df), data = data.raw,
+           family = poisson)
+       summ <- summary(fit)
+       summ.coef <- summ$coefficients["l1pm10tmean",
+           2]
+       c(coef(fit)["l1pm10tmean"], summ.coef)
+ })
```

Figure 6.7(b) shows the estimates of the log-relative risk for PM_{10} and mortality for Denver. The estimates for 2 df per year are very different for the natural spline model compared to the smoothing spline model. However, estimates for the range 4–14 df per year are all quite similar to those obtained via smoothing splines.

6.6.3 Choosing degrees of freedom from the data

So far we have shown the effect of varying the degrees of freedom in the smooth function of time on estimates of the log-relative risk of PM_{10} on mortality. Figure 6.7 suggests that estimates can vary dramatically by changing the degrees of freedom used. However, we have not indicated any way to choose how many degrees of freedom are appropriate. One possibility is to choose the estimate that we know to be least confounded based on prior scientific knowledge. But one might also want a method that allows the data to choose the appropriate amount of smoothness.

Numerous methods for choosing the amount of smoothness for the smooth function of time have been proposed in the literature. These methods generally fall into the categories:

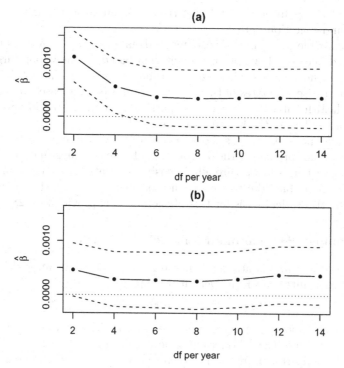

Fig. 6.7. Estimates of the log-relative risk for (solid circles) PM_{10} for Denver, Colorado, 1987–2000, as the number of degrees of freedom per year in the smooth function of time is varied, using (a) smoothing splines with asymptotically exact standard errors and (b) parametric natural cubic splines; dashed lines indicate approximate 95% confidence intervals.

1. Methods based on predicting the outcome variable (i.e., mortality)
2. Methods based on predicting the exposure variable (i.e., PM_{10})

Methods falling into category 1 include methods that choose a model based on minimizing the Akaike information criterion (AIC) or the Schwarz Bayes' information criterion (BIC), or minimizing residual autocorrelation via the partial autocorrelation function (PACF) or tests for white noise. The one thing these methods all have in common is that they minimize a criterion evaluated on models that are constructed to predict the outcome variable (mortality).

Methods falling into category 2 include those described in [28] and [76] whereby a criterion such as the generalized cross-validation (GCV) score or AIC is minimized over a set of models constructed to predict the exposure (PM_{10}). In [28] the authors showed this class of methods has the specific advantage that they will produce either unbiased or asymptotically unbiased estimates of the pollution log-relative risk, depending on the nature of the mortality and pollution data.

Although widespread in their use, methods falling into category 1 are generally flawed because they optimize a criterion based on the wrong target. In air pollution and health studies we are primarily interested in obtaining accurate and precise estimates of the association between increases in pollution levels and health outcomes. We are not particulately interested in developing a model for predicting the health outcome itself.

Therefore, methods such as those in category 1 which attempt to identify the best model for predicting the outcome, can fail in certain situations. In [76] Peng and coauthors showed through extensive simulation that these methods can produce more biased estimates than those based on predicting exposure. Much of the theoretical basis for this phenomenon is provided in [28].

6.6.4 Example: Semiparametric model for Detroit

We can briefly demonstrate the semiparametric modeling approach using PM_{10} and mortality data from Detroit, Michigan.

```
> data <- readCity("det", collapseAge = TRUE)
```

This approach chooses the degrees of freedom for the smoother by fitting a model that predicts the PM_{10} time series. This model fit will produce an estimate of the degrees of freedom that we can subsequently use in our health effects model which uses mortality as the outcome. To estimate the degrees of freedom for predicting the exposure PM_{10}, we use the bruto function in the **mda** package, which estimates the degrees of freedom via generalized cross-validation [44].

```
> library(mda)
> pm10 <- data$l1pm10tmean
> x <- unclass(data$date)
> use <- complete.cases(pm10, x)
> br.fit <- bruto(x[use], pm10[use])
> optimal.df <- br.fit$df
```

Here we can see that the estimated degrees of freedom is 39.1, or approximately 2.8 degrees of freedom for each of the 14 calendar years of data. Given the estimated degrees of freedom we can fit our health effects model using the gam function from the **gam** package. This function represents the smooth function of time as a smoothing spline.

```
> library(gam)
> fit <- gam(death ~ l1pm10tmean + s(date,
+     optimal.df), data = data, family = quasipoisson)
> v <- gam.exact(fit)
```

The estimate of the log-relative risk is

```
> print(v$coefficients["l1pm10tmean", "Estimate"])
```

```
[1] 0.000651555
```

and the asymptotically exact standard error is

```
> print(v$coefficients["l1pm10tmean", "A-exact SE"])
```

```
[1] 0.0001139625
```

The standard error computation is computed separately by the `gam.exact` function [28]. Because we used the `quasipoisson` family in the call to `gam`, we can check for the presence of overdispersion in the data by taking the `summary` of the fitted gam.

```
> summary(fit)$dispersion
```

```
quasipoisson
    1.160927
```

Here we see that the overdispersion is modest, which is common for mortality data [51].

Continuing this example, we can compare the approaches to choosing the degrees of freedom from categories 1 and 2. First we calculate the optimal degrees of freedom that best predicts the PM_{10} time series.

```
> pm10 <- data$l1pm10tmean
> x <- unclass(data$date)
> use <- complete.cases(pm10, x)
> br.fit <- bruto(x[use], pm10[use])
> df.pm10 <- br.fit$df
```

Then we calculate the optimal degrees of freedom for predicting the mortality time series.

```
> death <- data$death
> use <- complete.cases(death, x)
> br.fit <- bruto(x[use], death[use])
> df.death <- br.fit$df
```

Given the optimal degrees of freedom, we can fit a GAM to the mortality and PM_{10} data and obtain the corresponding log-relative risk estimates.

```
> fit1 <- gam(death ~ l1pm10tmean + s(date,
+       df.pm10), data = data, family = quasipoisson)
> fit2 <- gam(death ~ l1pm10tmean + s(date,
+       df.death), data = data, family = quasipoisson)
> v1 <- gam.exact(fit1)
> v2 <- gam.exact(fit2)
```

Table 6.3 shows the estimated percent increase in mortality for a 10 $\mu g/m^3$ increase in PM_{10}. We can see that the optimal degrees of freedom for predicting PM_{10} was about 2.8 degrees of freedom per year, which resulted in a risk estimate of a 0.65% increase in mortality with a 10 $\mu g/m^3$ increase in PM_{10}.

The optimal degrees of freedom for predicting mortality was 6 per year, resulting in a slightly higher risk estimate of a 0.74% increase in mortality for a 10 $\mu g/m^3$ change. Note that although there is a difference in the degrees of freedom chosen by the two methods, there is little difference in the standard errors obtained.

	Estimate	A-exact SE	df/year
Predict PM$_{10}$	0.65	0.11	2.79
Predict Mortality	0.74	0.11	6.05

Table 6.3. Comparison of methods for choosing the degrees of freedom in the smooth function of time

6.6.5 Smoothers

Common choices for representing the smooth function of time include natural splines, penalized splines, and smoothing splines. (Other less common choices are loess smoothers or sine/cosine functions.) The first is fully parametric, wherease the latter two may be considered more flexible. With natural splines, one constructs a spline basis with knots at fixed locations throughout the range of the data and the choice of knot locations can have a substantial impact on the resulting smooth. Smoothing splines and penalized splines circumvent the problem of choosing the knot locations by constructing a very large spline basis and then penalizing the spline coefficients to reduce the effective number of degrees of freedom. Smoothing splines place knots at every (unique) data point and are sometimes referred to as full-rank smoothers because the size of the spline basis is equal to the number of observations. Penalized splines, sometimes called low-rank smoothers, are more general in their definition in that both the size of the spline basis and the location of the knots can be specified. Low-rank smoothers can often afford significant computational benefits when applied to larger datasets such as those used here. A comprehensive treatment of the various spline methods can be found in [95].

In [76] the authors showed that although the choice of the smoother can alter the resulting estimates of the association between air pollution and health, the particular smoother used has much less of an impact than the choice of degrees of freedom used in the smoother. In the end, it is often advantageous to choose the smoother that is most convenient. What matters most is not "how you smooth" but rather "how much you smooth."

6.7 Multisite Studies: Putting It All Together

In this chapter we have focused on building a time series model for estimating the association between an exposure such as air pollution and an outcome such as mortality or hospitalization in a single site, city, or location. However, if we have data for multiple sites, then we would like to combine information from those multiple sites.

We can fit model (6.7) to each site for which we have data. Here we take the 20 largest cities (by population) in the NMMAPS database

```
> meta <- getMetaData("citycensus")
> ord <- order(meta[, "pop100"], decreasing = TRUE)
> sites <- as.character(meta[ord, "city"][1:20])
```

and independently compute estimates of the association between nonaccidental mortality and lag 1 PM_{10}, adjusting for temperature, age category, and a smooth function of time.

```
> r <- lapply(sites, function(site) {
+       sitedata <- readCity(site)
+       fit <- glm(death ~ l1pm10tmean + agecat +
+           tmpd + ns(date, 8 * 14), data = sitedata,
+           family = poisson)
+       summ <- summary(fit)
+       summ$coefficients["l1pm10tmean", c("Estimate",
+           "Std. Error")]
+ })
> results <- do.call("rbind", r)
```

Figure 6.8 shows a histogram of the estimates from the 20 cities. We can see that there is substantial range of variation in the estimates, ranging from -0.0001 to 0.0011.

The next chapter deals specifically with statistical methods for combining information across multiple sites and for handling any natural heterogeneity of estimates across sites. These methods include hierarchical models and Bayesian methods of estimation to account for the different sources of variability.

6.8 Summary

Estimating the health effects associated with short-term exposure to air pollution poses several statistical challenges. Most of these challenges arise because we are aiming at estimating a very small relative risk in the presence of several measured and unmeasured confounders. Semiparametric models are a very useful tool to adjust for measured confounders when the association between these confounders and the exposure and the outcome is likely to be nonlinear, as, for example, is the case with weather variables. Adjusting for these

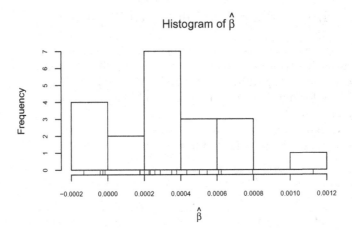

Fig. 6.8. Histogram of city–specific log-relative risk estimates from 20 NMMAPS cities, 1987–2000.

nonlinear effects is obtained by including a smooth function of each potential confounder in the regression model. Semiparametric models are also useful for estimating the air pollution risk by removing information at the timescales that are most likely to be affected by unmeasured confounders, such as seasonality and long-term trends. The information at longer timescales can be removed by including a smooth function of time with *df* degrees of freedom in the regression model.

The degrees of freedom *df* measures the degree of adjustment for confounding bias. Choosing *df* is itself a very challenging problem. In this chapter we have reviewed and compared several approaches that have been proposed in the literature to remove confounding bias. It is important here to make a clear distinction between prediction and estimation. Previous approaches in the literature have proposed selecting *df* to optimize prediction of the outcome. We argue that in time series studies of air pollution and health we have a different goal: we are interested in estimating an air pollution coefficient that has the smallest mean squared error. Thus, the choice of *df* requires a bias–variance tradeoff with respect to the estimation of the risk coefficient.

Choosing a large *df* leads to a very aggressive adjustment for unmeasured confounding. This will remove the bias, but also will remove most of the temporal variation in the residuals thus leading to a large variance of the estimated air pollution coefficient. Choosing a small *df* corresponds to a weak adjustment for unmeasured confounding. This might lead to bias but it will also provide a more precise estimate of the air pollution coefficient. Often the investigator has some prior knowledge of the timescales that are less likely to be affected by unmeasured confounding. Under this scenario, it is always good practice to show the sensitivity of the air pollution risk estimates to the choice of *df*.

6.9 Reproducibility Package

The **cacher** package associated with all of the analyses and figures in this chapter can be downloaded from the Reproducible Research Archive by running

```
> clonecache(id = "49c090223e7b16d72240a928f69bccd72a0a164c")
```

which will download all of the relevant code and data files.

6.10 Problems

To begin, we pose the following overall questions.

1. What variables/factors might confound the relationship between air pollution and mortality?
2. What happens to the PM_{10}-mortality relationship when we try to "adjust" for season and temperature? Is the relationship consistent across the various strata?
3. Are the estimates of the association between PM_{10} and mortality the same in each city? Why might they be different?

In the problems that follow, the goal is to estimate the risk of mortality associated with short-term exposure to air pollution adjusted for confounding by temperature and season. In order to remove the influences of potential confounders, we need to compare mortality when air pollution is higher to otherwise similar days where air pollution is lower. A key issue is how to define "similar".

One possibility is to match days based on the season or on temperature. For example, if we estimate the association between air pollution and mortality by restricting to days where the temperature is the same, then temperature cannot confound the relationship between air pollution and mortality. Similarly, if we stratify the analysis by season, then season cannot confound the relationship. Ultimately, the common approach for adjusting for confounding is to build regression models. In this part, we present some examples on how to adjust for temporal measured and unmeasured confounders in time series studies of air pollution and health.

1. We begin with some simple modeling. Use the `glm` function to fit a log-linear Poisson generalized linear model of all-cause nonaccidental mortality (death) versus PM_{10} exposure at lag 1 (`l1pm10tmean`). Do this for Chicago (`chic`), New York (`ny`), and Los Angeles (`la`).
2. For a given city's data frame, subset the data frame and create four separate data frames, one for each season/quarter of the year. To create a "winter" data frame for Chicago, you can do

```
load("chic.rda")
winter <- subset(chic, quarters(date) == "Q1")
```

Data frames for the other three seasons/quarters can be constructed in a similar fashion.

3. Fit four separate models of nonaccidental mortality versus lag 1 PM_{10} using the four season-specific data frames.

4. Fit a model of nonaccidental mortality and temperature (tmpd).

5. For each city, divide the temperature range into three categories: cold (tmpd < 50 degrees), warm ($50 \leq$ tmpd < 80), hot (tmpd $\geq$ 80). Create three new data frames by subsetting the city's data frame into separate cold, warm, and hot data frames. (Note: You might want to think up some other definitions of cold, warm and hot.)

6. Fit three separate models of death $\sim$ tmpd, one for each temperature range.

7. Fit three separate models of death $\sim$ l1pm10tmean, one for each temperature range.

8. Divide the data into $3 \times 4 = 12$ different temperature-by-season data frames and fit a model of death $\sim$ l1pm10tmean within each stratum.

9. Fill in the regression coefficient for l1pm10tmean associated with each pairwise combination in the following table for each city (Chicago, New York, LA):

	Winter	Spring	Summer	Fall
Cold				
Warm				
Hot				

For the PM_{10} coefficients, you may want to express them as the percent increase in mortality for a 10 $\mu g/m^3$ increase in PM_{10} (a standard reporting scale).

10. In the previous problems, some of the season $\times$ temperature categories have no data in them. This might cause a problem when you start looking at many variables at once. One compromise we can make to avoid this situation is to use a multiple regression model.

    Use the glm function to fit the overdispersed Poisson model (6.4) of nonaccidental mortality and lag 1 PM_{10} (death $\sim$ l1pm10tmean) for Chicago, New York, and Los Angeles.

11. Use the gam function from the **gam** package to fit the same model as above and use the gam.exact function to calculate the asymptotically exact standard error of the air pollution coefficient accounting for the smooth function of time. Compare the results you obtain using the gam function with those you obtain using the glm function.

12. Create two new categorical variables (factors), one named `season` corresponding to the four seasons/quarters and one named `temp` corresponding to three temperature ranges (cold, warm, hot). See what happens to the coefficient for `l1pm10tmean` when you add `season` and `temp` to the model.

13. Try adding other variables from the city's data frame to the model and see how the log-relative risk for `l1pm10tmean` changes.

14. Use the `glm()` and `gam()` function to fit the overdispersed Poisson models (6.4) of nonaccidental mortality and ozone (`o3tmean`) at lags 0, 1, 2, and 3 for Chicago, New York, and Los Angeles. You can use the `Lag` function from the **tsModel** package to fit a distributed lag model.

15. Use the `gam.exact` function to calculate the asymptotically exact standard error of the air pollution coefficient accounting for the smooth function of time.

16. For the ozone analysis, estimate the cumulative effect for lags 0 through 3.

17. Investigate the sensitivity of the single lag and cumulative effects to the inclusion of lagged temperature variables into the model.

18. Repeat the ozone analysis separately for the "warm" (April–September) and the "cold" seasons (October–March).

7

Pooling Risks Across Locations
and Quantifying Spatial Heterogeneity

7.1 Hierarchical Models for Multisite Time Series Studies of Air Pollution and Health

In this chapter we illustrate Bayesian hierarchical models for pooling health risk estimates across locations to produce regional and national average health risk estimates. We extend the modeling approaches for time series data for a single location in a hierarchical fashion to analyze multiple time series measured at several spatial locations. For example, consider a large study region A (e.g. United States), partitioned into subregions A^s, $s = 1, \ldots, S$ (e.g., zipcodes or counties), let Y_t^s be daily time series data of counts of a health outcome (e.g., daily number of deaths or hospital admissions), let x_t^s be the exposure to an environmental agent (e.g., air pollution levels measured from one or more monitoring stations), let z_t^s be other time-varying confounders (e.g., temperature and humidity), and let β^s be the true log-relative rate measuring temporal associations between Y_t^s and x_t^s adjusted by z_t^s in the subregion s.

The main goal of this chapter is to illustrate how to combine information across locations for estimating an overall association between daily variations in exposure and daily variations in the health outcome, by taking into account time-varying confounders and the variability across locations of the β^s. In addition, we show how borrowing strength across locations can provide better estimates of location-specific risks. To address these goals we describe Bayesian hierarchical models for spatial time series data that rely upon different assumptions on the spatial correlation of the β^s.

Bayesian hierarchical models provide an unified approach for combining evidence across locations, quantifying the sources of variability, and identifying effect modification [62, 71, 40, 12]. Hierarchical models have been familiar to statisticians for the last four decades. Because of the development of computational tools that facilitate their implementation [118, 43], they have been applied widely in many disciplines. Recently they have been applied to analysis of multisite time series data of air pollution and mortality [11, 53, 93, 35, 127, 108].

In the remainder of this chapter, we describe and compare three Bayesian hierarchical models for analyses of spatial time series data characterized by three different assumptions about the geographical heterogeneity (or spatial correlation) of the β^s. We apply these hierarchical models to the MCAPS dataset, described in Chapter 2.

We have applied the semiparametric Poisson regression model described in Chapter 6 to the daily time series (Y_t^s, x_t^s, z_t^s) for $s = 1, \ldots, 202$. Figure 7.1 shows maximum likelihood estimates and 95% confidence intervals of the log-relative risk of hospital admissions for heart failure $\hat{\beta}^s$.

```
> library(MCAPS)
> initMCAPS("MCAPS")
> mcaps <- getData("estimates.subset")
> r <- subset(mcaps, outcome == "heart failure")
> beta <- r$beta
> std <- sqrt(r$var)
> n <- length(beta)
> rng <- range(beta - 1.96 * std, beta +
+      1.96 * std)
> plot(beta, seq_len(n), xlim = rng, pch = 20,
+      xlab = expression(hat(beta)), ylab = "County")
> segments(beta - 1.96 * std, seq(n), beta +
+      1.96 * std, seq(n))
> abline(v = 0, lty = 2)
```

These estimates denote the percent increase in hospital admissions for heart failure associated with a 10 $\mu g/m^3$ increase in $PM_{2.5}$ at lag 0 in location s.

As you can see, there is large variability of the MLEs (127 are positive, 75 are negative). However, there is also a substantial overlap between the 95% confidence intervals. The primary statistical questions of interest are:

1. Is there evidence that short-term variations in $PM_{2.5}$ are associated with hospitalization risk for cardiovascular and respiratory disease on average across the nation?
2. Is this evidence the same across geographical regions?
3. Is it reasonable to pool these estimates across geographical locations to provide a national estimate of risks?

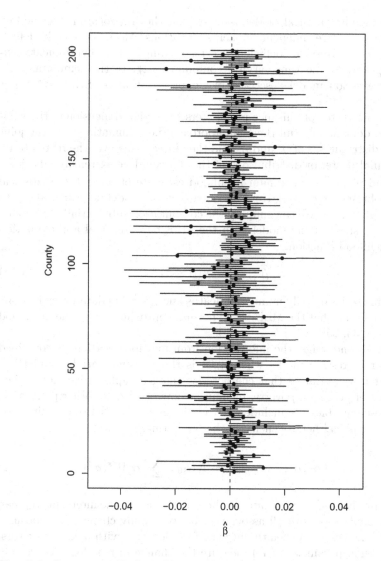

Fig. 7.1. County-specific log-relative risks for hospital admission for heart failure for 202 U.S. counties, 1999–2002.

7.1.1 Two-stage hierarchical model

The two-stage hierarchical model assumes that the true location-specific log-relative rates β^s are independent across locations. More specifically, let β^s and $\boldsymbol{\eta}^s$ be the regression coefficients corresponding to the environmental exposure x_t^s and to the time-varying confounders z_t^s, in the semiparametric Poisson regression model described in Chapter 6; that is, $E[Y_t^s \mid x_t^s, z_t^s] = \exp\left(\beta^s x_t^s + \boldsymbol{\eta}^s z_t^s\right)$.

When the vector of nuisance parameters $\boldsymbol{\eta}^s$ is high-dimensional, the computational demand of a full Bayesian approach (i.e., simulating from the joint posterior distributions of β^s and $\boldsymbol{\eta}^s$ and then integrating over the $\boldsymbol{\eta}^s$ to obtain the marginal posterior distributions of the β^s) could be extremely laborious. Let $\widehat{\beta}^s$ and v^s be the maximum likelihood estimate of β^s and its statistical variance obtained by fitting the Poisson regression model described above to the data (y_t^s, x_t^s, z_t^s). We can simplify the computation substantially by replacing the first stage of the model with the MLE-based normal approximation to the likelihood function:

$$\widehat{\beta}^s \mid \beta^s \sim N(\beta^s, v^s) \tag{7.1}$$

For time series of daily number of deaths and pollution data for eight years of data, we found that the MLE-based normal approximation to the likelihood is adequate [35, 25].

At the second stage, the information from multiple locations is combined in a linear regression model where (β^s) is the outcome variable and (W_j^s) are explanatory variables that characterize the geographical location s (i.e., percentage of people in poverty, median income, average of other pollutants, etc.). These variables are included in the hierarchical model to explain some of the geographical heterogeneity of the β^s. Formally:

$$\beta^s \mid \alpha_0, \alpha_1, \ldots, \alpha_p, \sigma^2 \sim N\left(\alpha_0 + \sum_{j=1}^{p} \alpha_j W_j^s, \sigma^2\right) \tag{7.2}$$

If the predictors W_j^s are centered about their means, the intercept (α_0) can be interpreted as the overall association between daily changes in exposures and daily changes in the health outcome for a location with mean predictors. The regression parameters (α_j) measure the change in true log-relative rate of mortality/morbidity associated with a unit change in the corresponding location-specific variable (W_j^s).

The sources of variation in the estimation of α_0 are specified by the levels of the hierarchical model. The variation of $\hat{\beta}^s$ about β^s is described by the within-location variance (v^s), which depends on the number of days with available exposure data, and on the predictive power of the location-specific regression model. The variation of β^s about α_0 is described by the between-location variance (σ^2) which measures the heterogeneity of the true log-relative rates across geographical locations unexplained by the covariates W_j^s.

The specification of a Bayesian hierarchical model (7.2) is completed with the selection of the prior distributions for the parameters at the top level of the hierarchy. If there is no desire to incorporate prior information into the analysis, then conjugate priors with large variances are a default choice. However, it is important to complete the Bayesian analysis by investigating the sensitivity of the substantive findings to the prior distributions.

In the two stage model without location-specific covariates, a point estimate of the overall effect α_0 can be obtained by taking a weighted average of the location-specific estimates $\widehat{\beta}^s$ with weights equal to $1/(v^s + \widehat{\sigma}^2)$ [20]. However, this approach relies upon a method of moments estimate of σ^2 and does not take into account the uncertainty of the estimate $\widehat{\sigma}^2$.

We can demonstrate the method of moments estimate by combining estimates of the short-term association between $PM_{2.5}$ and hospital admission for cerebrovascular disease in the MCAPS study.

```
> library(tsModel)
> library(MCAPS)
> mcaps <- getData("estimates.subset")
> r <- subset(mcaps, outcome == "cerebrovascular disease")
> p <- with(r, pooling(beta, var))
> print(p)
```

```
                  Estimate Std. Error t value
National avg. 0.00071573 0.00026438  2.7072
                   Pr(>|t|)
National avg. 0.003686 **
---
Signif. codes:  0 *** 0.001 ** 0.01 * 0.05 . 0.1   1
```

The method of moments estimate of the heterogeneity is

```
> print(p[["het"]])
```

```
[1] 0.001330954
```

The heterogeneity of the effects across locations is more completely assessed using a Bayesian approach. In fact the inspection of the posterior distribution of σ^2 provides a better characterization of the degree of heterogeneity of the effects across location than a point estimate of σ^2 and/or the classical χ^2 test of $\sigma^2 = 0$.

Posterior distributions of all parameters of interest specified in the two-stage can be estimated by using Markov chain Monte Carlo methods [119, 43]. Specifically, we use the computational algorithm by Everson and Morris [38] known as TLNISE to approximate the posterior distributions of all the unknown parameters.

Alternatively the two-stage hierarchical model 7.2 can be also fitted by use of Geobugs [115]. Note that in Geobugs it is straightforward to fit hierachical models with nonnormal random effect distributions such as the student-t and mixture of normal distributions.

7.1.2 Three-stage hierarchical model

The two-stage hierarchical approach described above can be extended to include additional levels of spatial aggregation (e.g., zip codes within cities, cities within counties, etc.) which lead to the estimation of additional sources of variability (within-location, between-location within region, and between regions), and potential effect modifiers at the location or regional level (see, e.g., Dominici et al. [25]).

Let $\widehat{\beta}_r^s$ and v_r^s be the relative rate estimate and the corresponding statistical variance for areas A^s nested within a larger geographical area A_r, where $\bigcup A_r = A$. At the first stage we assume that

$$\widehat{\beta}_r^s \mid \beta_r^s \sim N(\beta_r^s, v_r^s) \tag{7.3}$$

At the second stage, we describe the heterogeneity of the location-specific effects within the geographical area r by assuming:

$$\beta_r^s \mid \alpha_{0r}, \alpha_{1r}, \ldots, \alpha_{pr}, \tau^2 \sim N(\alpha_{0r} + \textstyle\sum_{j=1}^p \alpha_{jr} W_{jr}^s, \sigma^2) \; s = 1, \ldots, S_r \tag{7.4}$$

where $\beta_r^1, \ldots, \beta_r^{S_r}$ is the collection of true log-relative rates for the S^r locations nested within the geographical region r; W^ss are the location-specific covariates centered with respect to their mean value for the locations belonging to region r; α_{0r} is the overall log-relative rate for the geographical region r when all the covariates are centered at their mean values; α_{jr} measures the change in β_r^s per unit of change in the location-specific covariate W_{jr}^s; and σ^2 measures the heterogeneity of the β_r^ss within each region r unexplained by the covariates W_{jr}^s.

At the third level of the hierarchy, we model the variability of the regional log-relative rates of mortality/morbidity (α_{0r}) across regions; we assume:

$$\alpha_{0r} \mid \alpha_0, \tau^2 \sim N\left(\alpha_0, \tau^2\right) \tag{7.5}$$

Here α_0 is the overall relative rate, and τ^2 measures the variance of α_{0r} across regions.

The sources of variation in the estimation of α_0 are now specified by three levels of the hierarchical model. As in the two-stage random effect model, the variation of $\widehat{\beta}_r^s$ about β_r^s is described by the within-location variance (v_r^s), which depends on the number of days with available exposure data, and on the predictive power of the location-specific regression model. The variation of β_r^s about α_{0r} is described by the between-location within-region variance (σ^2). Finally, the variation of the α_{0r} about α_0 is described by the between-region variance (τ^2).

As an exploratory analysis, prior to fitting a full Bayesian hierarchical model, we can quantify the two sources of variations (within region and across regions) by running in R an analysis of variance applied to the MLEs $\hat{\beta}$.

```
> library(MCAPS)
> library(xtable)
> initMCAPS()
> est <- getData("estimates.subset")
> mcaps <- subset(est, outcome == "cerebrovascular disease")
> fit <- lm(beta ~ region7, data = mcaps,
+       weights = 1/var)
> summary(fit)

Call:
lm(formula = beta ~ region7, data = mcaps, weights = 1/var)

Residuals:
     Min        1Q    Median        3Q       Max
-3.27220 -0.65297   0.04316   0.64634   2.87122

Coefficients:
                    Estimate  Std. Error  t value
(Intercept)        -0.001997    0.001417   -1.410
region7Midwest      0.002420    0.001480    1.635
region7Northeast    0.003926    0.001492    2.631
region7Northwest    0.002682    0.002059    1.302
region7South        0.003602    0.001598    2.254
region7Southeast    0.002692    0.001543    1.744
region7West         0.001829    0.001491    1.227
                    Pr(>|t|)
(Intercept)          0.1602
region7Midwest       0.1037
region7Northeast     0.0092 **
region7Northwest     0.1943
region7South         0.0253 *
region7Southeast     0.0827 .
region7West          0.2213
---
Signif. codes:  0 *** 0.001 ** 0.01 * 0.05 . 0.1   1

Residual standard error: 1.049 on 195 degrees of freedom
Multiple R-squared: 0.07534,   Adjusted R-squared: 0.04689
F-statistic: 2.648 on 6 and 195 DF,  p-value: 0.01717
```

The region7 variable indicates in which of seven regions of the United States each county falls. One can see from the summary output that the region indicator explains a portion of the variation in the MLEs and its inclusion into the model is significant.

The specification of the model (7.5) is completed with the selection of the prior distributions for the parameters at the top level of the hierarchy. We assume a priori that these parameters are independent and we choose vague conjugate priors with large variances.

As for the hierarchical model (7.2), here we also used the TLNISE algorithm of Everson and Morris [38] to approximate the posterior distributions of all the unknown parameters separately within each geographical region. We first examine the estimates by the seven regions of the country.

```
> library(tlnise)

Two-level normal independent sampling
estimation (version 0.2-7)

> library(MCAPS)
> initMCAPS()
> options(scipen = 4)
> est <- getData("estimates.subset")
> mcaps <- subset(est, outcome == "cerebrovascular disease")
> region.ind <- model.matrix(~region7 -
+      1, mcaps)
> region7tlnise <- with(mcaps, {
+      initTLNise()
+      tlnise(beta, var, region.ind, intercept = FALSE,
+          prnt = FALSE, seed = 123, labelw = levels(region7))
+ })
> print(round(region7tlnise$gamma, 6))
                   est        se      est/se
Central    -0.001996 0.001443 -1.383668
Midwest     0.000425 0.000477  0.890275
Northeast   0.001924 0.000484  3.976672
Northwest   0.000628 0.001499  0.418726
South       0.001530 0.000762  2.006147
Southeast   0.000670 0.000622  1.076872
West       -0.000054 0.000601 -0.090466
```

We also examine the estimates when we divide the country into simply "east" and "west".

```
> est <- getData("estimates.subset")
> mcaps <- subset(est, outcome == "cerebrovascular disease")
> region.ind <- model.matrix(~regionEW -
+      1, mcaps)
> regionEWtlnise <- with(mcaps, {
+      initTLNise()
+      tlnise(beta, var, region.ind, intercept = FALSE,
+          prnt = FALSE, seed = 123, labelw = levels(regionEW))
+ })
> print(round(regionEWtlnise$gamma, 6))
            est       se      est/se
East   0.001112 0.000282  3.947410
West  -0.000222 0.000532 -0.416818
```

Alternatively we can fit model (7.5) as an unique hree-stage Bayesian hierarchical model using the Gibbs sampling.

7.1.3 Spatial correlation model

One limitation of the three-stage hierarchical model described above is that two locations s, s' far in terms of their geographical distance but belonging to the same geographical region r are considered "more similar" than two closer locations, but belonging to two separate geographical regions.

To overcome such limitation, we can relax the three-stage hierarchical model described above by the spatial correlation model [30]. Here we assume that each location-specific relative rate is shrunk toward the average relative rate in the neighboring locations, where neighboring locations are defined based on their geographical distance. More specifically, at the second stage of the hierarchical model, we assume that the β^s are normally distributed with a common mean $\alpha_0 + \sum_{j=1}^{p} \alpha_j W_j^s$, and variance σ^2. Differently from the two-stage hierarchical model described above where we assume that β^s and $\beta^{s'}$ are independent, here we express the degree of similarity of the log-relative rates in locations s and s' as function of the Euclidean distance between the cities. More specifically, we assume that:

$$\text{cor}(\beta^s, \beta^{s'}) = \exp(-\phi \times \text{distance between } s \text{ and } s'). \tag{7.6}$$

The parameter ϕ represents the rate of decay to zero of the correlation as the distance between the two locations increases. Of course, under this model formulation other types of distances can be considered as alternatives to the Euclidean distance. The parameter ϕ is typically unknown and estimated from the data.

The model specification is completed by assigning prior distributions to the unknown parameters. As with the two-stage hierarchical model, we can assign conjugate priors to the α parameters and to σ^2. More specifically, we can assume a priori that α has a Normal distribution with large variance and that σ^{-2} has a Gamma distribution with scale and shape parameters both equal to 0.001. Finally, one possible prior for the parameter ϕ is a uniform distribution in the range $[\phi_{\min}, \phi_{\max}]$. For example, the values $\phi_{\min}$ and $\phi_{\max}$ can be selected so that, if $\phi = \phi_{\min}$, the correlation between the two relative risks at the maximum distance between the locations is 0.01 and at the minimum distance between the locations is 0.8. If $\phi = \phi_{\max}$, the correlation between the two relative risks at the maximum distance between the locations is 0 and at the minimum distance between the locations is 0.5. Other ranges for ϕ are possible and choosing a reasonable range will depend on the specific dataset being used.

To approximate the posterior distributions of all the parameters of interest for the spatial correlation model, one can resort to simulation-based methods, and in particular the software alma in R [47] which is based on an adaptive Metropolis–Hastings algorithm [75]. We demonstrate a simpler approach below as an example of sensitivity analysis with respect to the correlation structure of the data.

We can perform sensitivity analyses of the estimate of the national average (α_0) with respect to modeling assumptions about heterogeneity and spatial correlation. In the three-stage model, we grouped the 202 counties (we excluded Honolulu and Anchorage from this analysis) into seven geographic regions (Northwest, Upper Midwest, Industrial Midwest, Northeast, Southern California, Southwest, Southeast). We assumed that city-specific estimates belonging to a particular region have a distribution with mean equal to the corresponding regional effect. This assumption implies that there exists regional heterogeneity: city-specific estimates of the air pollution effects are shrunk toward their regional means, and regional means are shrunk toward the national mean, respectively.

We can fit the data to a spatial correlation model, where we assume that each city-specific air pollution effect is shrunk toward the average air pollution effects in the neighboring cities, where neighboring cities are defined based on their geographical distance [21, 30, 27]. We use the correlation function in 7.6 to define the spatial structure and fit the model using the spatialgibbs function in the **tsModel** package. This function takes as inputs the relative rates for each location (along with their estimated variances), the x and y coordinates for each location, and a value for the parameter ϕ determining the strength of spatial correlation. We begin by obtaining the MCAPS relative rate estimates for the heart failure outcome and merge them with the latitude and longitude for each of the county locations.

```
> library(MCAPS)
> initMCAPS()
> est <- getData("estimates.subset")
> mcaps <- subset(est, outcome == "heart failure")
> locations <- read.csv("locations.csv",
+       colClasses = c("character", rep("numeric",
+           2)))
> mcaps <- merge(mcaps, locations, by = "fips")
```

We can then fit the spatial Bayesian hierarchical model using different values of ϕ to control the strength of spatial correlation. Here, we use values of ϕ as 1, 0.1, and 0.01, representing weak, moderate, and strong spatial correlation between neighboring relative rates. The $\phi = 1$ model is very close to an independence model wherease $\phi = 0.01$ allows counties that are very far apart to be correlated. For example, using $\phi = 0.01$, the two counties that are the farthest apart in this dataset are allowed to have a correlation of approximately 0.5.

```
> library(tsModel)
> g1 <- with(mcaps, spatialgibbs(beta, var,
+       long, lat, phi = 1))
> g0.1 <- with(mcaps, spatialgibbs(beta,
+       var, long, lat, phi = 0.1))
> g0.01 <- with(mcaps, spatialgibbs(beta,
+       var, long, lat, phi = 0.01))
```

Figure 7.2 shows the marginal posterior distributions of the national average effect under the three different spatial correlation models. The value

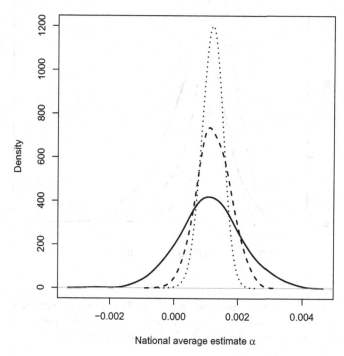

Fig. 7.2. Marginal posterior distributions of the overall effect   under the weak (dotted), moderate (dashed), and strong (solid) spatial correlation Bayesian hierarchical models for 202 U.S. counties, 1999–2002.

of the national average estimate (i.e., posterior mean) is robust to the different spatial models. As expected, the national average estimate under the strong correlation model shows a larger posterior interval than the national average estimate under the weak correlation model because of the assumed dependence between the estimates.

Figure 7.3 shows the posterior distributions of the heterogeneity parameter σ under the three different spatial models. Here we see that the mean of the distribution shifts as we assume more spatial correlation and the uncertainty increases. The posterior for the weak correlation model shows the weight of the evidence about the amount of heterogeneity and it gives the largest weights at values near zero indicating homogeneity or little heterogeneity. The larger posterior mean of the heterogeneity standard deviation under the moderate and strong correlation models reflects the assumption of larger total variance. More details of these types of analyses can be found in [26].

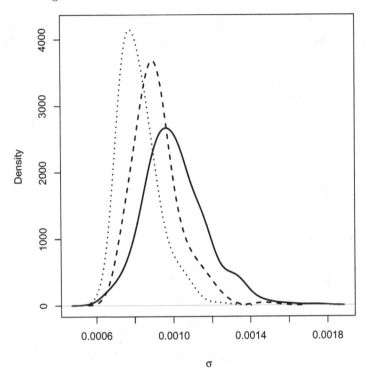

Fig. 7.3. Marginal posterior distributions of the heterogeneity parameter   under the weak (dotted), moderate (dashed), and strong (solid) spatial correlation Bayesian hierarchical models risks for 202 U.S. counties, 1999–2002.

7.1.4 Sensitivity analyses to the adjustment for confounders

We consider the following overdispersed Poisson semiparametric model used in the NMMAPS analyses

$$\log E[Y_t^c] = \text{age-specific intercepts} + \beta^c(\alpha)PM_{10t}^c + s(t, \alpha \text{ df/year}) + \\ + s(\text{temp}_t, 6) + s(\text{dewpoint}_t, 3) + \text{age} \times s(t, 1 \text{ df/year})$$

where y_t^c is the daily number of deaths in city c, PM_{10t} is the daily level of PM_{10}, temp and dew are the temperature and dewpoint temperature, and the age-specific intercepts correspond to the three age groups of younger than 65, between 65 and 75, and older than 75. Justification for the selection of the degrees of freedom to control for longer-term trends, seasonality and weather can be found in Samet et al. [100, 102, 98], Kelsall et al. [54], and Dominici et al. [35].

Based upon the statistical analyses of the 100 NMMAPS cities and additional exploratory analyses, we set α to take values $1, 2, \ldots, 20$. As in the previous model formulation, this choice allows the degree of adjustment for confounding factors to vary greatly.

We then assume the following two-stage Normal–Normal hierarchical model: Stage I: $\widehat{\beta}^c(\alpha) \sim N(\beta^c(\alpha), v^c(\alpha))$; Stage II: $\beta\ (\alpha) \sim N(\beta\ (\alpha), \tau^2(\alpha))$ where $\beta\ (\alpha)$ and $\tau^2(\alpha)$ are the national average air pollution effects and the variance across cities of the true city-specific air pollution effects, both as a function of α.

We fit the hierarchical model by using a Bayesian approach, with a flat prior on $\beta\ (\alpha)$ and uniform prior on the shrinkage factor $\tau^2(\alpha)/[\tau^2(\alpha) + v^c(\alpha)]$ [38]. Sensitivity of the national average estimates to the specification of the prior distribution of τ^2 has been explored elsewhere [25].

To investigate sensitivity of the national average estimates to model choice, for each value of α, we estimate $\widehat{\beta}^c(\alpha)$ and $v^c(\alpha)$ using three methods: (1) GAM with smoothing splines and approximated standard errors (GAM-approx s.e.); (2) GAM with smoothing splines and asymptotically exact standard errors (GAM-exact); and (3) GLM with natural cubic splines (GLM). Figure 7.4 shows the national average estimates (posterior means) as a function of α. Dots, octagons, and triangles denote estimates under GAM-exact, GAM-R, and GLM, respectively. The shaded region represents 95% posterior intervals of the national average estimates under GLM. Figure 7.4 provides

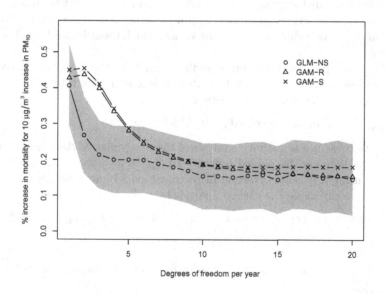

Fig. 7.4. Sensitivity analysis of the national average estimate of the percent increase in mortality for a 10 $\mu g/m^3$ increase in PM_{10} at lag 1. The three fitting methods used are GLM with natural cubic splines (GLM-NS), GAM with penalized splines (GAM-R), and GAM with smoothing splines (GAM-S). The shaded region shows the 95% posterior intervals for the estimates obtained using GLM-NS.

strong evidence for association between short-term exposure to PM_{10} and non-accidental mortality, which persists for different values of α. Consistent with the results for individual cities, the national average estimates decrease as α increase, and level off for α larger than 10 with a very modest increase in posterior variance.

This picture also shows robustness of the results to model choice (GAM versus GLM). National average estimates under GAM-exact are slightly smaller than those obtained under GAM-approx, although this difference is very small. These two sets of estimates are comparable because in hierarchical models, underestimation of standard errors at the first stage ($\sqrt{v^c(\alpha)}$) is compensated by the overestimation of the heterogeneity parameter at the second stage ($\tau^2(\alpha)$). Thus the posterior total variance of the national average estimates remains approximately constant [19].

7.2 Example: Examining Sensitivity to Prior Distributions

In this section we illustrate the use of the **cacher** package to reproduce some results from a multi-site time series study examining the short-term relationship between particulate matter $\leq 2.5\mu m$ in aerodynamic diameter ($PM_{2.5}$) and daily hospital admission rates for various cardiovascular and respiratory diseases [33].

This study produced a county-specific estimate of the log-relative risk relating increases in daily $PM_{2.5}$ with daily hospital admission rates. These risks can be found at the study's Web site at

http://www.biostat.jhsph.edu/MCAPS/

Below, we present a sensitivity analysis of these log-relative risks and demonstrate how they can be pooled together to obtain a "national average" risk estimate using a two-level Normal hierarchical model [more details in 35].

First, we can clone the cached analysis by calling clonecache.

```
> clonecache("http://www.biostat.jhsph.edu/rr/mcaps.cache")

created cache directory '.cache'
```

Here we see that there is only one source file available, the mcaps.R file.

```
> showfiles()

[1] "mcaps.R"

> sourcefile("mcaps.R")
```

We can list the code expressions with the code function.

```
> code(1:7)
```

```
source file: mcaps.R
1   Sys.setlocale(locale = "C")
2   estimates <- read.csv("http://www.biostat.jh...
3   estimates <- transform(estimates,
4   library(tlnise)
5   HF <- subset(estimates, outcome ==
6   initTLNise()
7   pooled <- with(HF, tlnise(beta,
```

The first six code expressions read the data from the Web site and pool the risk estimates for heart failure across the 202 counties in the study. For the pooling, we use Phil Everson's TLNISE software [38], an R version of which is available on CRAN. The first thing we can do is the verify that we are capable of producing the same results that the original authors did. The checkcode function can be used to check the first six expressions.

```
> checkcode(1:7)

evaluating expression 1
checking expression 2
+ object 'estimates' OK
checking expression 3
+ object 'estimates' OK
evaluating expression 4
checking expression 5
+ object 'HF' OK
evaluating expression 6
checking expression 7
+ object 'pooled' OK
```

Here we see that the six expressions were evaluated properly and the objects created matched those created by the original authors. Database objects were downloaded from the archive as needed.

The original pooled national average log-relative risk for hospitalization for heart failure can be found by loading the cached objects for expression 7.

```
> loadcache(7)
> pooled$gamma

         est           se    est/se
0 0.001291823 0.0002505152 5.156663
```

This risk estimate shown in the est column can be interpreted as a 1.29% increase in admissions of heart failure associated with a 10 $\mu g/m^3$ increase in ambient $PM_{2.5}$.

One important issue in this analysis is the sensitivity of the Bayesian hierarchical model to the specification of the prior distribution. In particular, the TLNISE software places a uniform prior on the second-level covariance matrix, sometimes referred to as the heterogeneity matrix, which describes the natural variation of the relative risks across counties. The original authors used the default settings, thus it is of interest to see if the national average estimates vary when this prior specification is altered.

The `tlnise` function has an option called `prior` which can be used to change the nature of the prior distribution on the second-level covariance matrix. Here we try two alternate priors. First, we need to call `loadcache` in order to obtain the data frame `HF`.

```
> loadcache(1:7)
> library(tlnise)
> p0 <- with(HF, tlnise(beta, var, prnt = FALSE,
+     prior = 0))
> p2 <- with(HF, tlnise(beta, var, prnt = FALSE,
+     prior = 2))
```

We can now compare the estimates obtained using the two alternative prior specifications with the original estimates

```
> rbind(p0$gamma, p2$gamma, pooled$gamma)

          est            se    est/se
0 0.001287913 0.0002499124  5.153457
0 0.001292679 0.0002501618  5.167373
0 0.001291823 0.0002505152  5.156663
```

Here we see that there is some variation between the estimates but the estimates are qualitatively similar.

7.3 Reproducibility Package

The full data and code for all of the analyses in this chapter (with the exception of the analysis done in Section 7.2) can be downloaded using the **cacher** package by running

```
> clonecache(id = "fd9f843bd5ad0b9e2265dacf1a8cda3fb813db50")
```

which will download the cached analysis from the Reproducible Research Archive.

7.4 Problems

1. Load the `estimates.subset` dataset from the **MCAPS** package. Plot the county-specific estimates of the relative rates for cerebrovascular disease and their approximate 95% confidence intervals.
2. Try plotting the same data but ranking the estimates from the largest to the smallest.
3. Apply the function `pooling` to estimate the national average and the heterogeneity parameter by using the method of moments. Interpret these two estimates.

4. Apply the function lm to estimate an average effect for each of the seven geographical regions.
5. Apply the function tlnise to estimate the national average and the heterogeneity parameter by using Bayesian computation methods. Compare these estimates with the ones obtained previously.
6. Do the same as the previous problem but separately for the counties located in the eastern and western United States.
7. Apply the function tlnise to all the outcomes and produce national average estimates and their 95% confidence intervals. Do you obtain the same results as the ones summarized in the Table 1 of the paper by Dominici et al. [33]?
8. Apply the function tlnise to the county-specific estimates (MLE) for cerebrovascular disease and obtain the Bayesian county-specific estimates (BE) and their 95% posterior intervals.
9. Plot side by side the MLE and the Bayesian estimates with their 95% uncertainty intervals versus county.
10. Rank the BE and their posterior intervals from the largest to the smallest estimate. Try to plot the ranked estimates and their 95% posterior intervals.
11. Plot the MLE county-specific estimates versus the county-specific characteristics found in the file countyinfo.rda.
12. Fit a weighted linear regression model having as dependent variable the county-specific MLE estimates and as independent variable each of the county-specific covariate. Weight the observation by 1 divided by the statistical variance of the MLEs.
13. You have provided evidence of significant adverse health effects that can occur from exposure to ambient levels of fine particulate matter $PM_{2.5}$ air pollution in a large nationwide sample of older adults. The breadth and size of their Medicare study population, and the recent EPA proposal for new legal limits for this air pollutant, raise a time-critical question:

    Can this study be used to further test the hypothesis that the EPA proposal to set a maximum daily exposure limit of 35 $\mu g/m^3$ will be sufficient to eliminate these adverse health effects?

    Conduct subset analyses to test whether this newly proposed air pollution standard, if achieved, could eliminate the public health risk of excess hospital admissions from exposures to $PM_{2.5}$ air pollution.

General questions to consider:

- Is there evidence that short-term variations in $PM_{2.5}$ are associated with hospitalization risk for cerebrovascular disease on average across the nation?
- Is this evidence the same across geographical regions and between the eastern and western United States? Is there evidence of heterogeneity across counties and geographical regions of the health effects of air pollution?

- Are counties with the largest health risks for $PM_{2.5}$ also the ones with largest average O_3 and NO_2? Can we identify county-specific characteristics that might explain why some counties have larger health risks than others?
- Are the relative risks estimates similar across cities? Is it reasonable to pool these estimates across geographical locations to provide a national estimate of risks? If yes, why? If no, why?
- Should we estimate health relative risks in Los Angeles by using data from Los Angeles only or should we also use data available in the other counties?
- What are the three cleanest counties in the United States (i.e., that have the smallest health risks associated with air pollution)? Should we move there? What are the three dirtiest counties in the United States? If you live in one of them, should you move out?

8

A Reproducible Seasonal Analysis
of Particulate Matter and Mortality
in the United States

8.1 Introduction

Multisite time series studies have provided strong evidence of a positive association between short-term variation in ambient levels of particulate matter (PM) and daily mortality counts [see, e.g., 88, 24, 7]. The models used in these studies have typically assumed that the association between PM and daily mortality is constant over the study interval. However, the short-term effects of PM on mortality might exhibit seasonal variation. Studies in a number of locations have shown that the characteristics of the PM mixture change throughout the year and that the relative and absolute contributions of particular components to PM mass may be different during different times of the year [37, Ch. 3 and references therein]. Patterns of human activity also change from season to season, so that a particular air pollution concentration in one season may lead to a different exposure in another season. Other potential time-varying confounding and modifying factors, such as temperature and influenza epidemics, can also affect estimates of short-term effects of air pollution on mortality differently in different seasons. All of the issues described above indicate a need to use alternative models for time series data on air pollution and health to incorporate time-varying pollution effects.

The composition of particulate matter is known to vary in the spatial domain as well, suggesting that seasonal patterns should be examined by geographical region [114]. For example, in the northwest United States, wood burning is a greater source of PM in the colder seasons than in the warmer months. The PM mixture in the eastern United States contains a large fraction of sulfates (almost 40% of total mass) originating from power plants in the Midwest, whereas PM in areas of the western United States such as Southern California and the Pacific Northwest contains more nitrates and organic compounds (approximately 30% of total mass) [114, 36, 37].

We can show the seasonal pattern of PM_{10} for different regions of the country. Here, we divide the United States into seven broad regions [see, e.g., 101] and show boxplots of the PM_{10} levels by season. We first need to load

the **NMMAPSdata** package [80] and obtain information about the cities in
the database. We have combined some of the city data in a single file that is
available from our Web site.

```
> library(NMMAPSdata)
> data(cities)
> baseURL <- "http://www.biostat.jhsph.edu/~rpeng/useRbook"
> load(url(file.path(baseURL, "CityDataCombined.rda")))
> cityList <- dget(file.path(baseURL, "cityList.R"))
```

We then need to extract the PM_{10} data from each city and split it by season
so that we can construct the boxplots for each of the regions. The PM_{10} data
in the NMMAPS database are detrended, with a smooth trend subtracted
out. In order to look at the absolute levels, we need to add the trend back in.

```
> pm10 <- with(citydata, pm10tmean + pm10mtrend)
> pmCity <- split(pm10, citydata$city)
> pmCity <- pmCity[names(pmCity) %in% cityList]
```

Using the season indicator variable in the dataset, we can split the PM_{10} data
by season. We also have a region indicator for each city, allowing us to further
split the data by region. There are seven regions used here, defined in the
original NMMAPS studies.

```
> SeasonIndicator <- citydata$Season[1:5114]
> regionID <- with(cities, region[match(cityList,
+     city)])
> regionNames <- c("Industrial Midwest",
+     "Northeast", "Northwest", "Southern California",
+     "Southeast", "Southwest", "Upper Midwest")
> pmSeas <- lapply(pmCity, split, f = SeasonIndicator)
> pmSeasRegion <- split(pmSeas, regionID)
> SeasonNames <- c("Winter", "Spring", "Summer",
+     "Fall")
> seasRegion <- lapply(pmSeasRegion, function(reg) {
+     l <- lapply(SeasonNames, function(seas) lapply(reg,
+         "[[", seas))
+     lapply(l, unlist)
+ })
```

Figure 8.1 shows the mean daily levels of PM_{10} by season for all cities
in each of the seven regions of the United States. The Southern California,
Northwest, and Southwest regions have their highest mean levels of PM_{10} in
the fall whereas other regions have their highest levels in the summer.

```
> par(mar = c(4, 5, 2, 0) + 0.1, las = 2)
> plot(0, 0, xlim = c(1, 35), ylim = c(0,
+     125), xaxt = "n", xlab = "Season",
+     ylab = expression(paste(PM[10], " level ",
+         bgroup("(", paste(mu, g/m^3),
+             ")")))), frame.plot = FALSE,
```

```
+       type = "n")
> for (i in seq(along = seasRegion)) {
+       y <- unlist(seasRegion[[i]])
+       n <- unlist(lapply(seasRegion[[i]],
+           length))
+       f <- factor(unlist(mapply(rep, seq(length(n)),
+           n)))
+       boxplot(y ~ f, outline = FALSE, add = TRUE,
+           at = seq(length(n)) + ((i - 1) *
+               5), pars = list(boxwex = 0.5),
+           lty = 1, axes = FALSE)
+ }
> axis(1, at = 1:35, labels = rep(c("Winter",
+       "Spring", "Summer", "Fall", NA), 7),
+       tick = FALSE, cex.axis = 0.7)
> text(seq(2.7, 35, 5), c(100, 100, 100,
+       120, 100, 100, 100), regionNames)
```

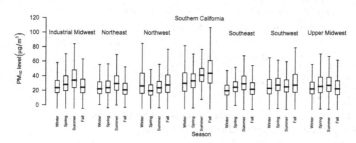

Fig. 8.1. Boxplots of regionally averaged daily levels of particulate matter less than 10 μm in aerodynamic diameter (PM$_{10}$) by season for 100 United States cities, 1987–2000.

Mortality and PM$_{10}$ levels are known to vary considerably across seasons. Generally, mortality tends to be higher in the winter and fall and lower in the summer and spring. To examine the seasonal variability of mortality in the NMMAPS dataset, we can look at mortality in the top ten largest cities according to the Census 2000 population.

```
> cityList <- with(cities, city[order(pop,
+       decreasing = TRUE)])[1:10]
> dCity <- with(citydata, split(death, city))
> dCity <- dCity[names(dCity) %in% cityList]
```

For each city, we split the mortality time series (death) by season

```
> SeasonIndicator <- citydata$Season[1:5114]
> dSeas <- lapply(dCity, split, f = SeasonIndicator)
```

and order the cities by decreasing population.

```
> ord <- order(with(cities, pop[match(names(dSeas),
+     city)]), decreasing = TRUE)
> dSeas <- dSeas[ord]
```

Figure 8.2 shows boxplots of the square root daily mortality counts for the largest ten cities in the United States, by season. Each city shows a clear decrease in mortality towards summer and a peak in the winter.

```
> par(mar = c(4, 4, 2, 0) + 0.1, las = 2)
> plot(0, 0, ylim = c(4, 17), xlim = c(1,
+     50), xlab = "Season", axes = FALSE,
+     ylab = "Square root daily mortality counts",
+     type = "n")
> for (i in seq(along = dSeas)) {
+     y <- unname(unlist(dSeas[[i]]))
+     n <- unname(unlist(lapply(dSeas[[i]],
+         length)))
+     f <- factor(unlist(mapply(rep, seq(length(n)),
+         n)))
+     boxplot(sqrt(y) ~ f, outline = FALSE,
+         add = TRUE, at = seq(length(n)) +
+             ((i - 1) * 5), pars = list(boxwex = 0.5),
+         lty = 1, axes = FALSE)
+ }
> SeasonNames <- c("Winter", "Spring", "Summer",
+     "Fall")
> axis(1, at = 1:50, labels = rep(c(SeasonNames,
+     NA), length(dSeas)), tick = FALSE,
+     cex.axis = 0.7)
> axis(2)
> par(las = 1)
> text(seq(2.5, 50, 5), c(8, 10, 8, 11,
+     10, 10, 10, 10, 10, 10), cityNames)
```

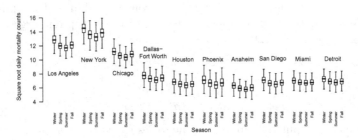

Fig. 8.2. Boxplots of square root daily mortality by season for the ten largest United States cities, 1987–2000.

In this chapter we outline some statistical methods for estimating seasonal patterns in the short-term effects of air pollution on mortality in multisite time series studies. We propose Bayesian semiparametric hierarchical models for estimating time-varying health effects within each city and for comparing temporal patterns across cities and geographical regions. Using data from the National Morbidity, Mortality, and Air Pollution Study (NMMAPS) [101], we estimate seasonal patterns in the short-term effects of PM less than 10 μm in aerodynamic diameter (PM$_{10}$) on daily nonaccidental mortality. The data have been extended from the original study to include 100 United States cities for the period 1987–2000, an addition of ten cities and six years of data. The seasonal patterns are estimated for seven geographical regions and on average for the entire United States. We explore the sensitivity of estimated seasonal patterns to temperature adjustment, copollutants, exposure lag, and adjustments for long-term mortality trends.

8.2 Methods

The NMMAPS database contains daily time series of mortality, weather, and air pollution assembled from publicly available sources for the largest 100 cities in the United States. A full description of the construction of the database can be found in [101]. The most recent data are available at http://www.ihapss.jhsph.edu/.

Within each city, we specify a semiparametric regression model for the time-varying log-relative rate using a generalized additive model framework [45]. More specifically, let Y_t^c be the total number of nonaccidental deaths on day t in city c. The Y_t^c are Poisson distributed with expectation μ_t^c and with possible overdispersion ϕ^c. The general form of the city-specific model is

$$
\begin{aligned}
Y_t^c &\sim \text{Poisson}(\mu_t^c) \\
\text{Var}(Y_t^c) &= \phi^c \mu_t^c \\
\log(\mu_t^c) &= \beta^c(t)\, x_{t-\ell}^c + \text{confounders}
\end{aligned}
\tag{8.1}
$$

where $x_{t-\ell}^c$ is the lag ℓ PM$_{10}$ level for day t.

The function $\beta^c(t)$ in Equation (8.1) represents the time-varying effect of PM$_{10}$ on mortality and is a yearly periodic function for estimating seasonal patterns. To estimate smooth seasonal patterns in the city-specific log relative rates, we use a sine/cosine model for $\beta^c(t)$ of the form

$$
\beta^c(t) = \beta_0^c + \beta_1^c \sin(2\pi t/365) + \beta_2^c \cos(2\pi t/365)
\tag{8.2}
$$

where β_0^c, β_1^c, β_2^c are estimated. In this model, the effect of PM$_{10}$ is allowed to vary smoothly over the course of a year, but is constrained to be periodic across years [e.g., 116]. Although it is possible to include higher-frequency basis terms for the representation of $\beta^c(t)$ in Equation (8.2), there is little reason to expect there to be much high-frequency variation in the seasonal effects of PM_{10}.

To allow for season-specific PM_{10} log-relative rates, we use a pollutant–season interaction model with indicator functions for each season:

$$\beta^c(t) = \beta^c_W \, I_{\text{winter}} + \beta^c_{Sp} \, I_{\text{spring}} + \beta^c_{Sm} \, I_{\text{summer}} + \beta^c_F \, I_{\text{fall}}, \qquad (8.3)$$

where winter, spring, summer, and fall are defined as beginning on December 21st, March 21st, June 21st, and September 21st, respectively. Although these seasonal estimates serve as concise summaries, it is unlikely that the effect of PM_{10} on mortality is discontinuous across seasons. Furthermore, the estimates depend on the specification of the season boundaries which are artificial and can differ considerably across geographic regions.

Our main effect model, which does not contain any adjustment for season takes $\beta^c(t)$ to be constant across time; that is,

$$\beta^c(t) = \beta^c. \qquad (8.4)$$

This model assumes a homogeneous log-linear effect of PM_{10} on mortality, a condition that was found appropriate in previous NMMAPS analyses [18, 31, 25, 26]. Note that the main effect model is nested within the interaction and sine/cosine models, so that if $\beta_W = \beta_{Sp} = \beta_{Sm} = \beta_F$ in Equation (8.3) and $\beta^c_1 = \beta^c_2 = 0$ in Equation (8.2), both models reduce to Equation (8.4).

The potential confounders included in equation 8.1 are similar to those used in previous NMMAPS analyses [e.g., 25, 26] and consist of indicators for the day of the week; age-specific intercepts corresponding to the categories of less than 65 years of age, 65–74 years, and 75 years or older; a smooth function of calendar time; and smooth functions of temperature and dewpoint temperature. In addition to the overall smooth function of time, two separate smooth functions of time are included for the older two age groups. All of the smooth functions are represented by natural cubic splines.

The complexity of each of the smooth functions of time and temperature is controlled by the numbers of degrees of freedom assigned to each function. We use seven degrees of freedom per year for the overall smooth function of time, which removes any fluctuations in mortality at timescales longer than two months. The separate smooth functions of time for the older two age categories each receive one degree of freedom per year to capture gradual trends specific to these age groups. For temperature we use six degrees of freedom and for dewpoint we use three degrees of freedom. A somewhat larger number of degrees of freedom is necessary for temperature in order to capture the well-known "J-shaped" nonlinear relationship between temperature and mortality. Others have adjusted for temperature simply by doing separate analyses of the data by season [70, 97, 35, 98, 99, 101].

All of the above models were fit using quasilikelihood methods as implemented in the R statistical software package [90]. The data are available via the **NMMAPSdata** package [80] and code for fitting the models is available on the Web at http://www.ihapss.jhsph.edu/data/NMMAPS/R/.

8.2.1 Combining information across cities

After fitting each of the city-specific models we use a hierarchical normal model for pooling information and borrowing strength across cities [see 99, 35, 25]. For a particular model, we have a city-specific maximum likelihood estimate $\widehat{\beta}^c$ which is a scalar for the main effect model in equation 8.4, a vector of length four for the pollutant-season interaction model in equation 8.3, and a vector of length three for the sine/cosine model in equation 8.2. $\widehat{\beta}^c$ is assumed to be normally distributed around the true city-specific log relative rates β^c with covariance matrix V^c, estimated within each city. In addition, the true rates are assumed to vary independently across cities according to a normal distribution, i.e.

$$\widehat{\beta}^c \mid \beta^c \sim \mathcal{N}(\beta^c, V^c)$$
$$\beta^c \mid \alpha, \Sigma \sim \mathcal{N}(Z^c \alpha, \Sigma) \tag{8.5}$$

where Σ is the covariance matrix describing the between-city variation of β^c and α is the overall mean for the cities. Z^c is a matrix of second-stage covariates for describing possible differences between cities. To characterize regional differences in seasonal patterns we include as a second-stage covariate an indicator for the following seven regions (also used in [101]): Industrial Midwest (19 cities), Northeast (17), Northwest (13), Southern California (7), Southeast (26), Southwest (10), and Upper Midwest (8).

The final national average estimate α represents the combined information from all of the cities. The diagonal elements of Σ measure the heterogeneity across cities and the off-diagonal elements represent the correlation of the estimates between cities. The hierarchical model is fit using the two level normal independent sampling estimation (TLNISE) software of [38] with uniform priors on α and Σ. This software provides a sample from the posterior distribution of Σ from which one can calculate posterior means and variances of the overall and city-specific pollution effects.

8.3 Results

The daily mortality counts for the years 1987–2000 include approximately 10 million deaths. By city, the daily average ranged from 2 deaths per day in Arlington, VA to 190 per day in New York, NY. The daily mean of PM_{10} ranged from 13 $\mu g/m^3$ in Coventry, RI to 49 $\mu g/m^3$ in Fresno, CA.

We would like to obtain national average estimates of the association between PM_{10} and daily mortality. These estimates incorporate all of the relevant data in the NMMAPS database and reflect the relevant uncertainties. In addition to nationally averaged estimates, we would like to obtain national estimates by season to see if there are any differences in the effects between seasons.

We begin by first fitting the city-specific models to the cities in the NMMAPS database.

```
> library(NMMAPSdata)
```

```
NMMAPS Data (version 0.4-3)
    Type citation("NMMAPSdata") for
    information on how to cite NMMAPSdata
    in publications.  Type ?NMMAPS for a
    brief introduction to the NMMAPS
    database.  Type vignette("NMMAPSdata")
    to view a short tutorial vignette.
```

```
> cityList <- dget(file.path(baseURL, "cityList.R"))
```

In this analysis we focus on using exposure lags of PM_{10} of 0, 1, and 2 days, so that lag 1 exposure indicates that we are comparing today's mortality with yesterday's PM_{10}.

```
> pollutants <- c("pm10tmean", "l1pm10tmean",
+     "l2pm10tmean")
```

We then loop over the cities and fit the models using the fitCitySeason function with the option season = "none". The results are stored in the list results.nonseasonal.

```
> library(splines)
> library(tsModel)
> results.nonseasonal <- vector("list",
+     length = length(pollutants))
> extractcoef <- function(x) summary(x)$coefficients
> extractors <- list(coefficients = extractcoef,
+     cov = vcov)
> for (i in seq(along = pollutants)) {
+     lag.results <- vector("list", length = length(cityList))
+     for (l in seq(along = cityList)) {
+         citydata <- readCity(cityList[l])
+         lag.results[[l]] <- try({
+             fitCitySeason(data = citydata,
+                 pollutant = pollutants[i],
+                 cause = "death", season = "none",
+                 extractors = extractors)
+         })
+     }
+     results.nonseasonal[[i]] <- lag.results
+ }
```

Once the nonseasonal city-specific models have been fit to all the cities for all three exposure lags, we can move on to fitting the pollutant–season interaction model. This process also makes use of the fitCitySeason function with the option season = "factor2" and stores the results in the list results.stepfun.

```
> results.stepfun <- vector("list", length=length(pollutants))
> for (i in seq(along = pollutants)) {
+     lag.results <- vector("list", length = length(cityList))
+     for (l in seq(along = cityList)) {
+         citydata <- readCity(cityList[l])
+         lag.results[[l]] <- try({
+             fitCitySeason(data = citydata,
+                 pollutant = pollutants[i],
+                 cause = "death", season = "factor2",
+                 extractors = extractors)
+         })
+     }
+     results.stepfun[[i]] <- lag.results
+ }
```

With the city-specific estimates from both the non-seasonal model and the pollutant–season interaction model, we can combined the estimates across cities using a two-level hierachical model. Specifically, we use the two-level Normal independent sampling estimation software of Everson and Morris [38]. We first combine the nonseasonal estimates

```
> library(tsModel)
> library(tlnise)

Two-level normal independent sampling
estimation (version 0.2-7)

> betacovTotal <- lapply(results.nonseasonal,
+     extractBetaCov, pollutant = "pm10")
> pooledTotal <- lapply(betacovTotal, poolCoef)
```

followed by the estimates from the pollutant-season interaction model.

```
> pooledSeas <- lapply(results.stepfun,
+     coefSeasonal, pollutant = "pm10",
+     method = "factor2")
> pooled <- lapply(seq(along = pooledSeas),
+     function(i) {
+         rbind(pooledSeas[[i]], pooledTotal[[i]])
+     })
```

The national average estimates of the overall and seasonal short-term effects of PM_{10} on mortality for lags 0, 1, and 2 are summarized in Table 8.1. Across all seasons, we found that the national average estimate of the effect of PM_{10} on mortality is largest at lag 1 and equal to an estimated 0.19 (95% posterior interval of 0.10, 0.28) percent increase in mortality per 10 $\mu g/m^3$ increase in PM_{10}. Previous NMMAPS analyses using data from the eight-year period 1987–1994 have reported similar slightly higher national average estimates for PM_{10} log relative rates [31, 26]. For example, the national average estimate reported in [26] was a 0.22 (0.03, 0.42) percent increase in mortality for a 10 $\mu g/m^3$ increase in PM_{10}. For PM_{10} at lag 1, the estimates for winter, spring, and fall are similar and equal to 0.15 $(-0.08, 0.39)$, 0.14 $(-0.14, 0.42)$, and 0.14 $(-0.06, 0.34)$, respectively. The estimate for summer is more than twice as large at 0.36 $(0.11, 0.61)$. PM_{10} at lag 0 appears to have a larger effect in the spring and much smaller effects in the other seasons. In addition, estimates for lag 0 have a much larger between-season difference (e.g., spring and winter) than those of lag 1. The estimates for lag 2 are generally smaller than those of lag 0 or 1 and, given the size of the posterior intervals, do not vary much across seasons.

In order to show smoothly varying estimates of the seasonal effects of PM_{10}, we fit the sine/cosine model to each city and combine the estimates across cities. Here, we use the fitCitySeason function with the option season = "periodic" and df.Season = 1 and store the results in the list results.smooth.

```
> library(tsModel)
> results.smooth <- vector("list", length = 3)
> for (k in seq(along = pollutants)) {
+      lag.results <- vector("list", length = length(cityList))
+      for (l in seq(along = cityList)) {
+          citydata <- readCity(cityList[l])
+          lag.results[[l]] <- try({
+              fitCitySeason(data = citydata,
+                  pollutant = pollutants[k],
+                  cause = "death", season = "periodic",
+                  df.Season = 1, extractors = extractors)
+          })
+      }
+      results.smooth[[k]] <- lag.results
+ }
```

Regional differences in the seasonal patterns of the PM_{10} relative rates were explored by including a region indicator variable in the second stage of the hierarchical model. For PM_{10} at lag 1, Figure 8.3 shows the results of estimating separate seasonal trends from the sine/cosine model for the seven regions of the United States. The Industrial Midwest and the Northeast have seasonal trends characterized as being lower in the winter and higher in the summer. In Southern California there is a larger effect (0.5 percent increase in mortality per 10 $\mu g/m^3$ increase in PM_{10}) that is constant all year. The effect of PM_{10} is close to zero all year round in the Northwest, Southeast, Southwest, and the Upper Midwest, but the Northwest experiences a slight increase during the summer months. With the exception of Southern California, all regions have a smaller effect in the winter months. Seasonal analyses for mortality due to cardiovascular and respiratory diseases (not shown) provided results that are qualitatively similar to those for total nonaccidental mortality, with larger summer effects in the Industrial Midwest and the Northeast regions, as well as overall for the entire United States.

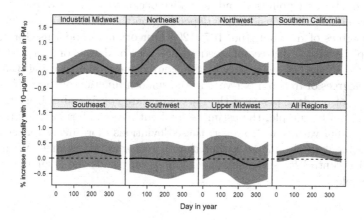

Fig. 8.3. National and regional smooth seasonal effects of PM_{10} (particulate matter less than 10 μm in aerodynamic diameter) at lag 1 for 100 U.S. cities, 1987–2000. Estimates were obtained by pooling city-specific coefficients from the sine/cosine model (Equation (8.2)). Dotted lines indicate pointwise 95% posterior intervals.

8.3.1 Sensitivity analyses

We performed several additional analyses to explore the sensitivity of the estimated seasonal PM_{10} log-relative rates to model specification. Specifically, we examined sensitivity to adjustment for long-term trends and seasonality in PM_{10} and mortality

```
> library(NMMAPSdata)
> library(splines)
> library(tsModel)
> cityList <- dget(file.path(baseURL, "cityList.R"))
> dfVec <- seq(3, 13, 2)
> extractcoef <- function(x) summary(x)$coefficients
> extractors <- list(coefficients = extractcoef,
+     cov = vcov)
> lagresults1 <- lapply(cityList, function(city) {
+     cityresults <- multiDFFit(dfVec, city,
+         pollutant = "l1pm10tmean", cause = "death",
+         season = "periodic", df.Season = 1,
+         extractors = extractors)
+     names(cityresults) <- paste("df",
+         dfVec, sep = "")
+     lapply(cityresults, postProcess)
+ })
```

Selecting the degrees of freedom of the smooth function of time used to control for long-term trends and seasonality is an important issue in time series models of air pollution and mortality because estimates of pollution co-efficients can change considerably depending on the specification of the number of degrees of freedom [106, 107, 120]. Our original model used a natural cubic spline with 7 degrees of freedom per year of data. For PM_{10} at lag 1, Figure 8.4 shows the sensitivity of the sine/cosine model to using 3, 5, 7, 9, and 11 degrees of freedom per year in the smooth function of time. With only 3 degrees of freedom per year the curves deviate considerably from those in Figure 8.3; for example, the estimate for Southern California exhibits much more seasonal variation. However, these deviations more likely reflect a lack of adjustment in the model rather than a real seasonal change. With more aggressive control for seasonality and long-term trends the estimates appear to be stable.

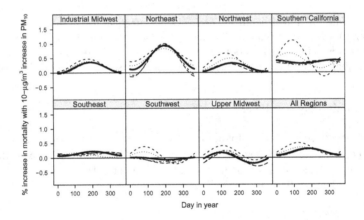

Fig. 8.4. Sensitivity of national and regional estimates of smooth seasonal effects for PM_{10} at lag 1 to the degrees of freedom assigned to the smooth function of time, 100 U.S. cities, 1987–2000. The degrees of freedom chosen were 3 (short dashed), 5 (dotted), 7 (solid), 9 (dot-dashed), and 11 (long dashed) degrees of freedom per year of data.

	Winter	Spring	Summer	Fall	All Seasons
Lag 0	-0.02 (-0.22, 0.17)	0.34 (0.08, 0.59)	0.13 (-0.12, 0.38)	0.05 (-0.16, 0.26)	0.09 (-0.01, 0.19)
Lag 1	0.14 (-0.09, 0.36)	0.16 (-0.13, 0.44)	0.34 (0.11, 0.57)	0.12 (-0.08, 0.32)	0.19 (0.09, 0.28)
Lag 2	0.11 (-0.11, 0.34)	0.04 (-0.23, 0.30)	-0.02 (-0.27, 0.23)	0.11 (-0.13, 0.35)	0.08 (-0.03, 0.19)

Table 8.1. National average estimates and 95% posterior intervals of the overall and season-specific effects of PM_{10} at lags 0, 1, and 2 for 100 cities, 1987–2000. Estimates were obtained by pooling city-specific coefficients from the main effect and pollutant–season interaction models, respectively, and represent the percent increase in daily mortality for a 10 $\mu g/m^3$ increase in PM_{10}.

8.4 Comments

In this chapter we have used a Bayesian semiparametric hierarchical model for estimating time-varying effects of air pollution on daily mortality. The model combines information across multiple cities to increase the precision of seasonal relative rate estimates. We found seasonal patterns for the national average effect of PM_{10} at both lag 0 and lag 1. Seasonal patterns appeared to vary by geographical region with a strong pattern for lag 1 appearing in the Northeast region. Equally interesting was the lack of seasonal variation in the southern regions of the country.

Understanding the health effects of PM components is an increasingly important research problem, as noted by the National Research Council [72]. Exploration of the spatial–temporal variation of the short-term effects of PM on mortality is essential to generating (or ruling out) specific hypotheses about the toxicity of PM components. Data are now available from the Environmental Protection Agency's $PM_{2.5}$ National Chemical Speciation Network which contain detailed time series information on the composition of $PM_{2.5}$. Knowledge of the spatial-temporal patterns of the short-term effects of PM will be necessary for guiding future analyses of these PM constituent data.

Regional differences in the short-term effects of PM_{10} were explored in NMMAPS [25, 26] and in the Air Pollution and Health: A European Approach (APHEA) study [52, 103]. Both studies found regional modification of the effect of PM_{10} on daily nonaccidental mortality. The results presented here are consistent with previous NMMAPS analyses with respect to regional average PM_{10} effects. The estimated seasonal patterns for lag 1 appear to have two distinct shapes. The Industrial Midwest, Northeast, and Northwest regions all exhibit a larger effect during the summer months wherease the other regions exhibit little seasonal variation. These patterns are somewhat sensitive to the lag of pollution used. Therefore, an important question is how the total effect of PM_{10} in a distributed lag model would vary by season. Unfortunately, the United States pollution database has daily PM levels for a small fraction of cities making it difficult to answer this question.

The results of this analysis admit several competing hypotheses. First, the PM constituents may vary by season in these regions with the most toxic particles having a spring/summer maximum. A detailed analysis of the regional and seasonal variation in PM constituents is needed to better understand these patterns. Second, even if the constituents do not vary substantially, it is possible that the higher short-term effect of ambient exposure to PM estimated in spring and summer in the Northeast regions could be the result of more time spent outdoors and therefore less exposure measurement error. A third possibility is that the particle effect may be swamped by the more powerful effect of winter infectious diseases so that it can only be observed when infectious diseases are less prevalent. This hypothesis does not explain the absence of a PM_{10} mortality association in the southern regions where infectious disease incidence is also seasonal. Finally, this result may reflect seasonally varying bias from an, as yet, unidentified source. Having established the pattern of regional and seasonal variation in the PM_{10} log-relative rate, a more targeted investigation of possible sources of such bias is now possible.

8.5 Reproducibility Package

Some of the code for producing the analyses in this Chapter has not been shown for the sake of brevity. The full data and code for all of the analyses and figures can be downloaded using the **cacher** package by calling

```
> clonecache(id = "6887df7ae339c24c39eaf6b491871fef7518b72f")
```

which will download the cached analysis from the Reproducible Research Archive. Some of the analyses in this Chapter, such as fitting the city-specific models to all of the NMMAPS cities are quite time-consuming and on first examination the reader might benefit from loading those results directly from the database rather than trying to reproduce them.

References

[1] H. Austin, W. D. Flanders, and K. J. Rothman. Bias arising in case–control studies from selection of controls from overlapping groups. *Int J Epidemiol*, 18:713–716, 1989.

[2] A. G. Barnett, G. M. Williams, J. Schwartz, T. L. Best, A. H. Neller, A. L. Petroeschevsky, and R. W. Simpson. The effects of air pollution on hospitalizations for cardiovascular disease in elderly people in Australian and New Zealand cities. *Environ Health Perspect*, 114(7):1018–1023, Jul 2006.

[3] A. G. Barnett, G. M. Williams, J. Schwartz, A. H. Neller, T. L. Best, A. L. Petroeschevsky, and R. W. Simpson. Air pollution and child respiratory health: a case-crossover study in Australia and New Zealand. *Am J Respir Crit Care Med*, 171(11):1272–1278, Jun 2005.

[4] T. F. Bateson and J. Schwartz. Control for seasonal variation and time trend in case–crossover studies of acute effects of environmental exposures. *Epidemiology*, 10:539–544, 1999.

[5] T. F. Bateson and J. Schwartz. Selection bias and confounding in case-crossover analyses of environmental time-series data. *Epidemiology*, 12:654–661, 2001.

[6] M. L. Bell, A. McDermott, S. L. Zeger, J. M. Samet, and F. Dominici. Ozone and short-term mortality in 95 US urban communities, 1987-2000. *J the Am Med Assoc*, 292(19):2372–2378, November 2004.

[7] M. L. Bell, J. M. Samet, and F. Dominici. Time-series studies of particulate matter. *Ann Rev Public Health*, 25:247–280, 2004.

[8] N. E. Breslow and N. E. Day. Statistical methods in cancer research. volume i - the analysis of case-control studies. In *IARC Scientific Publication Series, No 32*. Internatina; Agency for Research on Cancer: Lyon, 1980.

[9] J. Buckheit and D. L. Donoho. Wavelab and reproducible research. In A. Antoniadis, editor, *Wavelets and Statistics*. Springer-Verlag, New York, 1995.

[10] A. Buja, T. Hastie, and R. Tibshirani. Linear smoothers and additive models. *Ann Statistics*, 17(2):453–555, 1989.

[11] R. Burnett and D. Krewski. Air pollution effects of hospital admission rates: A random effects modelling approach. *Canadian J Statistics*, 22:441–458, 1994.

[12] B. P. Carlin and T. A. Louis. *Bayes and Empirical Bayes Methods for Data Analysis*. Chapman &; Hall, New York, 1996.

[13] C. Chatfield. *The Analysis of Times Series: An Introduction*. Chapman & Hall/CRC, 5th edition, 1996.

[14] D. Clayton and M. Hills. *Statistical Models in Epidemiology*. Oxford University Press, 1993.

[15] R. B. Cleveland, W. S. Cleveland, J. E. McRae, and I. Terpenning. STL: A seasonal-trend decomposition procedure based on loess. *J Official Statist*, 6:3–73, 1990.

[16] D. R. Cox and D. O. Oakes. *Analysis of Survival Data*. Chapman & Hall, 1984.

[17] F. C. Curriero, K. S. Heiner, J. M. Samet, S. L. Zeger, L. Strug, and J. A. Patz. Temperature and mortality in 11 cities of the eastern United States. *Am J Epidemiol*, 155:80–87, 2002.

[18] M. J. Daniels, F. Dominici, J. M. Samet, and S. L. Zeger. Estimating particulate matter-mortality dose-response curves and threshold levels: An analysis of daily time-series for the 20 largest us cities. *Am J Epidemiol*, 152(5):397–406, 2000.

[19] M. J. Daniels, F. Dominici, and S. L. Zeger. Understimation of standard errors in multi-site time series studies. *Epidemiology*, 15(1):57–62, 2004.

[20] R. DerSimonian and N. Laird. Meta-analysis in clinical trials. *Control Clin Trials*, 7:177–188, 1986.

[21] P. Diggle, R. Moyeed, and J. Tawn. Model-based geostatistics. *Appl Stat*, 47:559–573, 1998.

[22] D. D'Ippoliti, F. Forastiere, C. Ancona, N. Agabiti, D. Fusco, P. Michelozzi, and C. A. Perucci. Air pollution and myocardial infarction in Rome: a case-crossover analysis. *Epidemiology*, 14(5):528–535, Sep 2003.

[23] D. Dockery, C. A. Pope, X. Xu, J. Spengler, J. Ware, M. Fay, B. Ferris, and F. Speizer. An association between air pollution and mortality in six U.S. cities. *N Engl J Med*, 329:1753–1759, 1993.

[24] D. W. Dockery and C. A. Pope. Epidemiology of acute health effects: Summary of time-series studies. In R. Wilson and J. Spengler, editors, *Particles in Our Air*, pages 123–147. Harvard University Press, 1996.

[25] F. Dominici, M. Daniels, S. L. Zeger, and J. M. Samet. Air pollution and mortality: Estimating regional and national dose-response relationships. *J Am Statist Assoc*, 97:100–111, 2002.

[26] F. Dominici, A. McDermott, M. Daniels, S. L. Zeger, and J. M. Samet. Mortality among residents of 90 cities. In *Revised Analyses of Time-Series Studies of Air Pollution and Health*, pages 9–24. The Health Effects Institute, Cambridge, MA, 2003.

[27] F. Dominici, A. McDermott, M. Daniels, S. L. Zeger, and J. M. Samet. *A Special Report to the Health Effects Institute on the Revised Analyses of the NMMAPS II Data*. The Health Effects Institute, Cambridge, MA., 2003.

[28] F. Dominici, A. McDermott, and T. Hastie. Improved semiparametric time series models of air pollution and mortality. *J Am Statist Assoc*, 99(468):938–948, 2004.

[29] F. Dominici, A. McDermott, S. L. Zeger, and J. M. Samet. Airborne particulate matter and mortality: Time-scale effects in four US cities. *Am J Epidemiol*, 157:1053–1063, 2002.

[30] F. Dominici, A. McDermott, S. L. Zeger, and J. M. Samet. National Maps of the Effects of PM on Mortality: Exploring Geographical Variation. *Environ Health Perspect*, 111:39–43, 2002.

[31] F. Dominici, A. McDermott, S. L. Zeger, and J. M. Samet. On the use of generalized additive models in time-series studies of air pollution and health. *Am J Epidemiol*, 156(3):193–203, 2002.

[32] F. Dominici, A. McDermott, S. L. Zeger, and J. M. Samet. Airborne particulate matter and mortality: timescale effects in four US cities. *Am J Epidemiol*, 157(12):1055–1065, Jun 2003.

[33] F. Dominici, R. D. Peng, M. L. Bell, L. Pham, A. McDermott, S. L. Zeger, and J. M. Samet. Fine particulate air pollution and hospital admission for cardiovascular and respiratory diseases. *J the Am Med Assoc*, 295(10):1127–1134, 2006.

[34] F. Dominici, R. D. Peng, S. L. Zeger, R. H. White, and J. M. Samet. Particulate air pollution and mortality in the United States: did the risks change from 1987 to 2000? *Am J Epidemiol*, 166(8):880–888, Oct 2007.

[35] F. Dominici, J. M. Samet, and S. L. Zeger. Combining evidence on air pollution and daily mortality from the twenty largest US cities: A hierarchical modeling strategy (with discussion). *J Royal Statist Soc, Ser A*, 163:263–302, 2000.

[36] Environmental Protection Agency. *Air Quality Criteria for Particulate Matter*. EPA/600/P-95/001aF. Office of Research and Development, Washington DC, 1996.

[37] Environmental Protection Agency. *Air Quality Criteria for Particulate Matter (Fourth External Review Draft)*. EPA/600/P-99/002aD and bD. Office of Research and Development, National Center for Environmental Assessment, Research Triangle Park, NC, 2003.

[38] P. J. Everson and C. N. Morris. Inference for multivariate normal hierarchical models. *J Royal Statist Soc, Ser B*, 62:399–412, 2000.

[39] W. J. Gauderman, R. McConnell, F. Gilliland, S. London, D. Thomas, E. Avol, H. Vora, K. Berhane, E. B. Rappaport, F. Lurmann, H. G. Margolis, and J. Peters. Association between air pollution and lung function growth in southern california children. *Am J Resp Crit Care Med*, 162:1383–1390, 2000.

[40] A. Gelman, J. Carlin, H. Stern, and D. Rubin. *Bayesian Data Analysis*. Chapman and Hall, London, 1995.

[41] R. Gentleman. Reproducible research: A bioinformatics case study. *Statist Appl Genetics Molec Biol*, 4(1):Article 2, 2005.

[42] R. C. Gentleman, V. J. Carey, D. M. Bates, B. Bolstad, M. Dettling, S. Dudoit, B. Ellis, L. Gautier, Y. Ge, J. Gentry, K. Hornik, T. Hothorn, W. Huber, S. Iacus, R. Irizarry, F. Leisch, C. Li, M. Maechler, A. J. Rossini, G. Sawitzki, C. Smith, G. Smyth, L. Tierney, J. Y. H. Yang, and J. Zhang. Bioconductor: open software development for computational biology and bioinformatics. *Genome Biology*, 5(10):R80, 2004.

[43] W. R. Gilks, S. Richardson, and D. J. Spiegelhalter, editors. *Markov Chain Monte Carlo in Practice*. Chapman & Hall/CRC, London, 1996.

[44] C. Gu. *Smoothing Spline ANOVA Models*. Springer, New York, 2002.

[45] T. J. Hastie and R. Tibshirani. *Generalized Additive Models*. New York: Chapman and Hall, 1990.

[46] Health Effects Institute. *Revised Analyses of Time-Series Studies of Air Pollution and Health. Special Report*. Health Effects Institute, Boston MA, 2003.

[47] R. Ihaka and R. Gentleman. R: A language for data analysis and graphics. *J Comput Graph Statist*, 5(3):299–314, 1996.

[48] J. J. K. Jaakkola. Case-crossover design in air pollution epidemiology. *Eur Respir J Suppl*, 40:81s–85s, May 2003.

[49] H. Janes, L. Sheppard, and T. Lumley. Case-crossover analyses of air pollution exposure data: referent selection strategies and their implications for bias. *Epidemiology*, 16(6):717–726, Nov 2005.

[50] H. Janes, L. Sheppard, and T. Lumley. Overlap bias in the case-crossover design, with application to air pollution exposures. *Stat Med*, 24(2):285–300, Jan 2005.

[51] P. Jordan, D. Brubacher, S. Tsugane, Y. Tsubono, K. Gey, and U. Moser. Modelling of mortality data from a multi-centre study in Japan by means of Poisson regression with error in variables. *Int J Epidemiol*, 26(3):501–507, 1997.

[52] K. Katsouyanni, G. Touloumi, E. Samoli, A. Gryparis, A. LeTertre, Y. Monopolis, G. Rossi, D. Zmirou, F. Ballester, A. Boumghar, and H. R. Anderson. Confounding and effect modification in the short-term effects of ambient particles on total mortality: Results from 29 European cities within the APHEA2 project. *Epidemiology*, 12:521–531, 2001.

[53] K. Katsouyanni, G. Touloumi, C. Spix, F. Balducci, S. Medina, G. Rossi, B. Wojtyniak, J. Sunyer, L. Bacharova, J. Schouten, A. Ponka, and H. R. Anderson. Short term effects of ambient sulphur dioxide and particulate matter on mortality in 12 European cities: Results from time series data from the APHEA project. *Brit Med J*, 314:1658–1663, 1997.

[54] J. E. Kelsall, J. M. Samet, S. L. Zeger, and J. Xu. Air pollution and mortality in Philadelphia, 1974–1988. *Am J Epidemiol*, 146(9):750–762, 1997.

[55] D. Krewski, R. T. Burnett, M. S. Goldberg, K. Hoover, J. Siemiatycki, M. Abrahamowicz, and W. H. White. Validation of the Harvard Six Cities Study of particulate air pollution and mortality. *N Engl J Med*, 350(2):198–199, Jan 2004.

[56] D. Krewski, R. T. Burnett, M. S. Goldberg, K. Hoover, J. Siemiatycki, M. Jerrett, M. Abrahamowicz, and W. H. White. *Reanalysis of the Harvard Six Cities Study and the American Cancer Society Study of Particulate Air Pollution and Mortality*. Cambridge, MA: Health Effects Institute, 2000.

[57] F. Laden, L. M. Neas, D. W. Dockery, and J. Schwartz. Association of fine particulate matter from different sources with daily mortality in six U.S. cities. *Environ Health Perspect*, 108(10):941–947, Oct 2000.

[58] F. Laden, J. Schwartz, F. E. Speizer, and D. W. Dockery. Reduction in fine particulate air pollution and mortality: Extendeladen2006d follow-up of the Harvard Six Cities study. *Am J Resp Crit Care Med*, 173(6):667–672, Mar 2006.

[59] C. Laine, S. N. Goodman, M. E. Griswold, and H. C. Sox. Reproducible research: Moving toward research the public can really trust. *Ann Intern Med*, 146:450–453, 2007.

[60] D. Levy, T. Lumley, L. Sheppard, J. Kaufman, and H. Checkoway. Referent selection in case–crossover analyses for acute health effects of air pollution. *Epidemiology*, 12:186–192, 2001.

[61] D. Levy, L. Sheppard, H. Checkoway, J. Kaufman, T. Lumley, J. Koenig, and D. Siscovick. A case-crossover analysis of particulate matter air pollution and out-of-hospital primary cardiac arrest. *Epidemiology*, 12: 193–199, 2001.

[62] D. V. Lindley and A. F. M. Smith. Bayes estimates for the linear model (with discussion). *J Royal Statist Soc, Ser B*, 34:1–41, 1972.

[63] Y. Lu and S. L. Zeger. On the equivalence of case-crossover and time series methods in environmental epidemiology. *Biostatistics*, 8(2): 337–344, Apr 2007.

[64] T. Lumley and D. Levy. Bias in the case–crossover design: implications for studies of air pollution. *Environmetrics*, 11:689–704, 2000.

[65] M. Maclure. The case–crossover design: A method for studying transient effects on the risk of acute events. *Am J Epidemiol*, 133:144–153, 1991.

[66] M. Maclure and M. A. Mittleman. Should we use a case-crossover design? *Ann Rev Public Health*, 21:193–221, 2000.

[67] B. D. Marx and P. H. C. Eilers. Direct generalized additive modeling with penalized likelihood. *Comput Statist Data Anal*, 28:193–209, 1998.

[68] P. McCullagh and J. A. Nelder. *Generalized Linear Models*. Chapman and Hall, 1989.

[69] M. Medina-Ramn, A. Zanobetti, and J. Schwartz. The effect of ozone and PM10 on hospital admissions for pneumonia and chronic obstructive pulmonary disease: a national multicity study. *Am J Epidemiol*, 163(6):579–588, Mar 2006.

[70] S. H. Moolgavkar, E. G. Luebeck, T. A. Hall, and et al. Air pollution and daily mortality in philadelphia. *Epidemiology*, 6(5):476–484, 1995.

[71] C. N. Morris and S.-L. Normand. Hierarchical models for combining information and for meta-analysis. pages 321–344, 1992.

[72] National Research Council. *Research Priorities for Airborne Particulate Matter: IV. Continuing Research Progress*. National Research Council of the National Academies, 2004.

[73] W. Navidi. Bidirectional case–crossover designs for exposures with time trends. *Biometrics*, 54:596–605, 1998.

[74] L. M. Neas, J. Schwartz, and D. Dockery. A case-crossover analysis of air pollution and mortality in Philadelphia. *Environ Health Perspect*, 107:629–631, 1999.

[75] G. Parmigiani and G. Huerta-Gomez. Adaptive Metropolis Hastings. Technical report, Johns Hopkins University, Baltimore MD, 2001.

[76] R. D. Peng, F. Dominici, and T. A. Louis. Model choice in time series studies of air pollution and mortality (with discussion). *J Royal Statist Soc, Ser A*, 169(2):179–203, 2006.

[77] R. D. Peng, F. Dominici, R. Pastor-Barriuso, S. L. Zeger, and J. M. Samet. Seasonal analyses of air pollution and mortality in 100 US cities. *Am J Epidemiol*, 161(6):585–594, Mar 2005.

[78] R. D. Peng, F. Dominici, and S. L. Zeger. Reproducible epidemiologic research. *Am J Epidemiol*, 163(9):783–789, 2006. doi:10.1093/aje/kwj093.

[79] R. D. Peng and S. P. Eckel. Distributed reproducible research using cached computations. Technical Report 147, Johns Hopkins University Department of Biostatistics, 2007. http://www.bepress.com/jhubiostat/paper147/.

[80] R. D. Peng and L. J. Welty. The NMMAPSdata package. *R News*, 4(2):10–14, September 2004.

[81] A. Peters, D. W. Dockery, J. E. Muller, and M. A. Mittleman. Increased particulate air pollution and the triggering of myocardical infarction. *Circulation*, 103:2810–2810, 2001.

[82] A. Peters, S. von Klot, M. Heier, I. Trentinaglia, A. Hrmann, H. E. Wichmann, H. Lwel, and C. H. R. in the Region of Augsburg Study Group. Exposure to traffic and the onset of myocardial infarction. *N Engl J Med*, 351(17):1721–1730, Oct 2004.

[83] J. M. Peters, E. Avol, W. J. Gauderman, W. Navidi, S. J. London, H. Margolis, E. Rappaport, H. Vora, H. Gong, Jr., and D. C. Thomas. A study of twelve southern california communities with differing levels and types of air pollution: Ii. effects on pulmonary function. *Am J Resp Crit Care Med*, 159:768–775, 1999.

[84] J. M. Peters, E. Avol, W. Navidi, S. J. London, W. J. Gauderman, F. Lurmann, W. S. Linn, H. Margolis, E. Rappaport, H. Gong, Jr., and D. C. Thomas. A study of twelve southern california communities with differing levels and types of air pollution: I. prevalence of respiratory morbidity. *Am J Resp Crit Care Med*, 159:760–767, 1999.

[85] C. A. Pope. Mortality effects of longer term exposures to fine particulate air pollution: review of recent epidemiological evidence. *Inhal Toxicol*, 19 Suppl 1:33–38, 2007.

[86] C. A. Pope, R. T. Burnett, M. J. Thun, E. Calle, D. Krewski, K. Ito, and G. D. Thurston. Lung cancer, cardiopulmonary mortality, and long-term exposure to fine particulate air pollution. *J the Am Med Assoc*, 287(9):1132–1141, 2002.

[87] C. A. Pope, R. T. Burnett, G. D. Thurston, M. J. Thun, E. E. Calle, D. Krewski, and J. J. Godleski. Cardiovascular mortality and long-term exposure to particulate air pollution: epidemiological evidence of general pathophysiological pathways of disease. *Circulation*, 109(1):71–77, Jan 2004.

[88] C. A. Pope, D. W. Dockery, and J. Schwartz. Review of epidemiological evidence of health effects of particulate air pollution. *Inhal Toxicol*, 7:1–18, 1995.

[89] C. A. Pope, M. Thun, M. Namboodiri, D. Dockery, J. Evans, F. Speizer, and C. Heath. Particulate air pollution as a predictor of mortality in a prospective study of U.S. adults. *Am J Resp Crit Care Med*, 151: 669–674, 1995.

[90] R Development Core Team. *R: A Language and Environment for Statistical Computing*. R Foundation for Statistical Computing, Vienna, Austria, 2004. ISBN 3-900051-00-3.

[91] T. Ramsay, R. Burnett, and D. Krewski. The effect of concurvity in generalized additive models linking mortality and ambient air pollution. *Epidemiology*, 14:18–23, 2003.

[92] J. Rice. Convergence rates for partially splined models. *Statist and Probab Lett*, 4:203–208, 1986.

[93] W. Roemer, G. Hoek, B. Brunekreef, A. Kalandidi, and J. Pekkanen. Daily variations in air pollution and respiratory health in a multicenter study: the peace project. *Eur Respir J*, 12:1354–1361, 1998.

[94] A. Rossini and F. Leisch. Literate statistical practice. In K. Hornik and F. Leisch, editors, *Proceedings of the 2nd International Workshop on Distributed Statistical Computing*, pages 1–10, 2003.

[95] D. Ruppert, M. P. Wand, and R. J. Carroll. *Semiparametric Regression*. Cambridge University Press, 2003.

[96] M. Ruschhaupt, W. Huber, A. Poustka, and U. Mansmann. A compendium to ensure computational reproducibility in high-dimensional classification tasks. *Statist Appl Genetics Molec Biol*, 3(1):Article 37, 2004.

[97] J. Samet, S. Zeger, J. Kelsall, J. Xu, and L. Kalkstein. Does weather confound or modify the association of particulate air pollution with mortality? *Environ Res, Sec A*, 77:9–19, 1998.

[98] J. M. Samet, F. Dominici, F. C. Curriero, I. Coursac, and S. L. Zeger. Fine particulate air pollution and mortality in 20 US cities. *N Engl J Med*, 343:1742–1749, 2000.

[99] J. M. Samet, F. Dominici, S. L. Zeger, J. Schwartz, and D. W. Dockery. *The National Morbidity, Mortality, and Air Pollution Study, Part I: Methods and Methodological Issues.* Health Effects Institute, Cambridge MA, 2000.

[100] J. M. Samet, S. L. Zeger, and K. Berhane. *The Association of Mortality and Particulate Air Pollution.* Health Effects Institute, Cambridge, MA., 1995.

[101] J. M. Samet, S. L. Zeger, F. Dominici, F. Curriero, I. Coursac, D. W. Dockery, J. Schwartz, and A. Zanobetti. *The National Morbidity, Mortality, and Air Pollution Study, Part II: Morbidity and Mortality from Air Pollution in the United States.* Health Effects Institute, Cambridge, MA., 2000.

[102] J. M. Samet, S. L. Zeger, J. Kelsall, J. Xu, and L. Kalkstein. *Air pollution, weather and mortality in Philadelphia, In Particulate Air Pollution and Daily Mortality: Analyses of the Effects of Weather and Multiple Air Pollutants. The Phase IB report of the Particle Epidemiology Evaluation Project.* Health Effects Institute, Cambridge, MA., 1997.

[103] E. Samoli, J. Schwartz, B. Wojtyniak, G. Touloumi, C. Spix, F. Balducci, S. Medina, G. Rossi, J. Sunyer, L. Bacharova, H. R. Anderson, and K. Katsouyanni. Investigating regional differences in short-term effects of air pollution on daily mortality in the APHEA project: A sensitivity analysis for controlling long-term trends and seasonality. *Environ Health Perspect*, 109(4):349–353, 2001.

[104] G. Sawitzki. Keeping statistics alive in documents. *J Comput Graph Statist*, 17:65–88, 2002.

[105] J. J. Schlesselman. *Case Control Studies: Design, Conduct, Analysis.* Oxford University Press, New York, 1994.

[106] J. Schwartz. Nonparametric smoothing in the analysis of air pollution and respiratory illness. *Canadian J of Statist*, 22:471–488, 1994.

[107] J. Schwartz. Total suspended particulate matter and daily mortality in Cincinnati, Ohio. *Environ Health Perspect*, 102(2):186–189, 1994.

[108] J. Schwartz. The distributed lag between air pollution and daily deaths. *Epidemiology*, 11(3):320–326, 2000.

[109] J. Schwartz. Harvesting and long term exposure effects in the relation between air pollution and mortality. *Am J Epidemiol*, 151:440–448, 2000.

[110] J. Schwartz. Is there harvesting in the association of airborne particles with daily deaths and hospital admission? *Epidemiology*, 12:55–61, 2001.

[111] J. Schwartz and J. T. Lee. Reanalysis of the effects if air pollution on daily mortality in seoul, korea: A case-crossover design. *Environ Health Perspect*, 107:633–636, 1999.

[112] J. Schwartz, A. Zanobetti, and T. Bateson. Morbidity and mortality among elderly residents of cities with daily PM measurements. In *Revised Analyses of Time-Series Studies of Air Pollution and Health*, pages 25–58. Health Effects Institute, Cambridge MA, 2003.

[113] P. Speckman. Kernel smoothing in partial linear models. *J Royal Statist Soc, Ser B*, 50(3):413–436, 1988.

[114] J. Spengler and R. Wilson. Emissions, dispersion, and concentration of particles. In R. Wilson and J. Spengler, editors, *Particles in Our Air*, pages 41–62. Harvard University Press, 1996.

[115] D. Spiegelhalter, A. Thomas, N. Best, and W. Gilks. *BUGS: Bayesian inference using Gibbs Sampler, version 0.30*. Cambridge, 1994.

[116] A. M. Stolwijk, H. Straatman, and G. A. Zielhuis. Studying seasonality by using sine and cosine functions in regression analysis. *J Epidemiol Community Health*, 53(4):235–238, 1999.

[117] J. M. Symons, L. Wang, E. Guallar, E. Howell, F. Dominici, M. Schwab, B. A. Ange, J. Samet, J. Ondov, D. Harrison, and A. Geyh. A case-crossover study of fine particulate matter air pollution and onset of congestive heart failure symptom exacerbation leading to hospitalization. *Am J Epidemiol*, 164(5):421–433, Sep 2006.

[118] A. Thomas, D. J. Spiegelhalter, and W. R. Gilks. Bugs: A program to perform Bayesian inference using Gibbs sampling. In *Bayesian Statistics 4. Proceedings of the Fourth Valencia International Meeting*, pages 837–842. Clarendon Press: Oxford, 1992.

[119] L. Tierney. Markov chains for exploring posterior distributions (with discussion). *Ann Statistics*, 22:1701–1762, Dec. 1994.

[120] G. Touloumi, R. Atkinson, A. Le Tertre, E. Samoli, J. Schwartz, C. Schindler, J. Vonk, G. Rossi, M. Saez, D. Rabszenko, and K. Katsouyanni. Analysis of health outcome time series data in epidemiological studies. *Environmetrics*, 15:101–117, 2004.

[121] S. Vedal. Ambient particles and health: Lines that divide. *J Air Waste Manage Assoc*, 47:551–581, 1996.

[122] J. C. Wakefield and R. E. Salway. A statistical framework for ecological and aggregate studies. *J Royal Statist Soc, Ser A*, 164:119–137, 2001.

[123] L. J. Welty and S. L. Zeger. Are the acute effects of PM_{10} on mortality in NMMAPS the result of inadequate control for weather and season? A sensitivity analysis using flexible distributed lag models. *Am J Epidemiol*, 162:80–88, 2005.

[124] S. N. Wood. Modelling and smoothing parameter estimation with multiple quadratic penalties. *J Royal Statist Soc, Ser B*, 62(2):413–428, 2000.

[125] A. Zanobetti et al. The temporal pattern of mortality responses to air pollution: a multicity assessment of mortality displacement. *Epidemiology*, 13:87–93, 2002.

[126] A. Zanobetti and J. Schwartz. The effect of particulate air pollution on emergency admissions for myocardial infarction: a multicity case-crossover analysis. *Environ Health Perspect*, 113(8):978–982, Aug 2005.

[127] A. Zanobetti, J. Schwartz, and D. Dockery. Airborne particles are a risk factor for hospital admissions for heart and lung disease. *Environ Health Perspect*, 108:1071–1077, 2000.

[128] A. Zanobetti, M. Wand, J. Schwartz, and L. Ryan. Generalized additive distributed lag models: quantifying mortality displacement. *Biostatistics*, 1:279–292, 2000.

[129] S. L. Zeger, F. Dominici, and J. M. Samet. Harvesting-resistant estimates of pollution effects on mortality. *Epidemiology*, 89:171–175, 1999.

Index

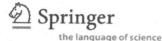

Springer
the language of science

springer.com

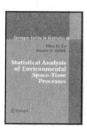

Statistical Analysis of Environmental Space-Time Processes

Nhu D. Le and James V. Zidek

This book provides a broad introduction to the subject of environmental space-time processes, addressing the role of uncertainty. It covers a spectrum of technical matters from measurement to environmental epidemiology to risk assessment. It showcases non-stationary vector-valued processes, while treating stationarity as a special case. In particular, with members of their research group the authors developed within a hierarchical Bayesian framework, the new statistical approaches presented in the book for analyzing, modeling, and monitoring environmental spatio-temporal processes.

2006. 341 pp. (Springer Series in Statistics) Hardcover
ISBN 978-0-387-26209-3

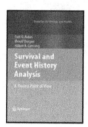

Survival and Event History Analysis
A Point Process View

Odd Aalen, Ørnulf Borgan, and Håkon Gjessing

The aim of this book is to bridge the gap between standard textbook models and a range of models where the dynamic structure of the data manifests itself fully. The common denominator of such models is stochastic processes. The authors show how counting processes, martingales, and stochastic integrals fit very nicely with censored data. Beginning with standard analyses such as Kaplan-Meier plots and Cox regression, the presentation progresses to the additive hazard model and recurrent event data.

2008. Approx. 550 pp. (Statistics for Biology and Health) Hardcover
ISBN 978-0-387-20287-7

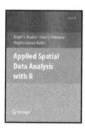

Applied Spatial Data Analysis with R

Roger S. Bivand, Edzer J. Pebesma, and Virgilio Gómez-Rubio

This book is divided into two basic parts, the first presenting R packages, functions, classes and methods for handling spatial data. The second part showcases more specialised kinds of spatial data analysis, including spatial point pattern analysis, interpolation and geostatistics, areal data analysis and disease mapping. The coverage of methods of spatial data analysis ranges from standard techniques to new developments, and the examples used are largely taken from the spatial statistics literature. All the examples can be run using R contributed packages available from the CRAN website, with code and additional data sets from the book's own website.

2008. Approx 400 pp. (Use R!) Softcover
ISBN 978-0-387-78170-9

Easy Ways to Order▶ Call: Toll-Free 1-800-SPRINGER • E-mail: orders-ny@springer.com • Write: Springer, Dept. S8113, PO Box 2485, Secaucus, NJ 07096-2485 • Visit: Your local scientific bookstore or urge your librarian to order.